The
Real
DOC
MARTIN

The Real DOC MARTIN

A MEMOIR

DR MARTIN STAGG

First published in Great Britain in 2024 by
Martin Stagg, in partnership with whitefox publishing

www.wearewhitefox.com

Copyright © Martin Stagg, 2024

ISBN 978-1-915635-85-3
Also available as an eBook
ISBN 978-1-915635-86-0

Designed and typeset by seagulls.net
Cover design by Madeline Meckiffe
Project management by whitefox
Printed and bound by CPI Group (UK) Ltd,
Croydon CR0 4YY

To the friends and family who encouraged me to write,
and must now accept some responsibility

Last Words

'Thank God you're here, doctor,' Jack said, standing up from his armchair.

Without another word, he fell to the floor, where he remained, unmoving. I swore under my breath and then quickly knelt down by his side and checked for his pulse and any breathing efforts.

None.

I tried to resuscitate him, but with no initial discernible effect. I was twenty-eight and not long out of my hospital medical training posts so was fairly confident and familiar with resuscitation techniques, and I also still carried some suitable injectable drugs in my visit bag, some of which I used then. I looked around in the living room but could not see a phone, so carried on trying a bit longer.

No response.

I left him for a few moments to see if there was a phone in the hall.

There wasn't.

I did not have a mobile phone as they were not widely available, nor affordable, at that time in the late 1980s. The dilemma was whether to continue trying to resuscitate this poor chap or whether to go to one of his neighbours' houses to seek out a phone in order to call an ambulance. I decided to stay with him and persevere. Eventually, after more than half an hour, I decided I had to abandon my attempts. All hope was gone, but I needed to inform others.

I went out of the house and back to the road and I looked up and down the street. No cars, other than mine, were parked there. There were no curtains twitching. I could see a telephone post with wires going to some nearby houses, further up the road, so I targeted those. I knocked on three different doors before somebody answered. There, I was allowed to use the phone. I rang 999 and requested an ambulance as well as the police, as there was a statutory duty to inform them of all unexpected deaths.

I walked back down the hill, obviously still upset and feeling fairly useless. As I approached the house to await the ambulance and police, I saw another man walking up the path to the front door. The son, George, I presumed. I stopped him and explained who I was, and confirmed who he was. I didn't want him to walk in and see his dad, unexpectedly and undignified in death. What followed was an excruciatingly awful few minutes as I explained the events of the last hour, including my failed attempts to save his dad.

He eyed me suspiciously, as you would, but appeared to accept my story. I told him that I was so sorry. We both went into the living room and sat down, the son on his dad's armchair, me on the sofa. His dad lay on the floor. Around him was some of the evidence of my failed resuscitation: a plastic airway, some syringes and drug vials, and paper wrappers for both. George wondered if we should tidy up, but I explained that it was better to leave things as they were for when the police arrived. I explained to him that his dad's death would be regarded as an unexpected death and there would need to be a coroner's inquest. I'm not sure that this further information helped him much at that stage.

The ambulance crew and policeman arrived quite quickly, and within a few moments of each other. The crew stayed with Jack and George while the police officer briefly interviewed me in the kitchen. He next spoke to George, and surveyed the scene in the living room, and then allowed the crew to take Jack's body away. He was to be taken to the local hospital morgue, where he would later have a post-mortem (PM). I was also authorised to leave, but before doing so I spoke to George once more, express-ing again how sorry I was about his dad's death.

The day had started out quite well, as it happens. I was in my first year working as a GP partner in Ashton-under-Lyne, East Manchester. It was to be my half-day off and I was excited as I had tickets to attend a Paul McCartney concert in Birming-ham. The plan was to finish morning surgery and visits, for me to then pick up my friend, Simon, from his house, and drive down to the Arena.

It was a very busy morning as we had two partners on leave and another one off with illness. I finished my surgery and walked into reception to the visit book in order to share out the home visits. There were nine. I then found out there were no other GP partners visiting that morning, so I expected to share these with the locum. I thought I would be generous and offer to do the larger share of the visits. That's when I found out about the locum's unavailability to help with the visits. He was unable to do any at all after his surgery because his car was being serviced; his wife had dropped him off earlier. Nine visits was an awful lot to do between surgeries, but at least I didn't have to get back for an afternoon clinic, although I still planned to drive to Birmingham, of course. For context, this was at least three more than I would normally ever do after a morning surgery, although I had often done more during full on-call day at week-ends or on bank holidays.

I'd set off with nine patient-record files and a rough route plan in my mind. It was a damp and dreary January day. My usual visiting order was to call on the patients who lived nearer the surgery first and then head outwards in a spiral. We had quite a wide catchment area at that time, so the latter visits were often twenty minutes' drive apart.

Two and a half hours after setting off, I'd headed towards the last visit, which was to an elderly gentleman, Jack. His son,

George, had complained to the receptionist that his father had 'a bad chest' when he'd rung to request a visit for him. I'd noticed that Jack had very thin medical records, suggesting he had been an infrequent attendee at the surgery. He had not consulted anyone recently and I had never seen him. His house was on a hill in a neat estate in an adjoining town some three miles from the surgery. I had parked up and opened the lattice gate and walked to the front door. When I'd knocked there had been no reply.

I'd knocked again. That time I'd heard a distant and muffled, 'Come in!' I'd opened the front door into a small hallway. The door into the front room was open so I'd walked in, just in time to hear Jack's final words.

Aftermath

After leaving Jack's, I drove straight to Simon's house, about two miles away. I was still a bit shaken up and thinking about the poor man and his son. I wondered if things could have turned out differently had I visited him earlier. I cringed inwardly and felt embarrassed and ashamed at both the failure to save him and the wretched revelation to his son. Dealing with death, and also breaking bad news, is an expected and fairly regular part of being a doctor generally, and a general practitioner particularly. The circumstances of the afternoon seemed far worse than usual, though. I suppose this was in part due to the lack of any immediate support, and the loss of control and dignity.

Simon listened to my story and made some supportive comments. He had bought sandwiches and snacks for our trip to Birmingham, all of which we ate there and then. After a few coffees we decided to try to catch the concert, and we made it with five minutes to spare. A memorable concert, I expect, although not for me, as I can barely remember anything about it at all. That doesn't really matter, and I have seen Macca in concert a number of times anyway, before and since.

More importantly, however, is that I have never forgotten Jack's sudden, sad death earlier that day, nor the sheer awfulness of the circumstances for him and his family. It was not the first death I had attended outside the hospital, but it was the first at which I was alone, and unable to summon any help.

Nowadays we all take mobile phones and other instant communications for granted, but back in the eighties, many people did not even have a home phone. I am not convinced that summoning an emergency ambulance would have necessarily saved Jack, but he would certainly have had a better chance than with me alone.

How had I got to that position? Being present and unable to prevent that sudden death and then having to explain it to a shocked family member? Being a GP is quite a responsible position, of course, and I had taken up that post at the age of twenty-seven. I was still fresh-faced enough, at that time, to be frequently told by patients that I 'look(ed) too young to be a doctor'.

I must have looked even more inappropriately youthful when I first qualified and worked as a hospital doctor, aged twenty-three. Most of the junior doctors did, and still do, of course. All of them have a different story of their route towards qualifying as a doctor, and then a different career path afterwards. I will tell you about mine here, in *The Real Doc Martin*, but first a few words about my namesake.

The Other Doc Martin

I have to admit to not fully enjoying all aspects of the *Doc Martin* TV series when it first appeared on ITV in 2004. I thought that the main actors were brilliant and I loved the beautiful filming locations. I also enjoyed 'guess the diagnosis' when the patients presented with unusual symptoms, which Martin usually picked up on fairly easily.

The problems I had with it initially were, firstly, accepting the premise that he had failed in his surgical career because of his phobia to blood. Many people have an initial distaste or phobia for blood when they are first exposed to an excess of it during their medical training and career but this invariably wears off with time, partly through familiarity and partly because one has to concentrate on the patient: being responsible for their care, and life. There also seemed to be an implication that there would be no exposure to blood in the new branch of his career. Again not true, although a GP would hopefully expect to see far less fresh red blood on a daily basis than a general surgeon would.

The second problem I had was the easy transition that he was able to make from a surgical to a General Practice career without any of the statutory training and examinations required in the real world.

Lastly, I could not believe that he had escaped being struck off every week, for his repeated rudeness and also breaches in confidentiality. I think that viewers like to see rudeness given back to rude people on TV, but most of these examples would still lead to a complaint in real life. Rude people also have rights and are less shy in exercising them than the rest of us, often when they have no genuine complaint.

What changed? I got over myself and stopped being so uptight, learning instead to relax into enjoying it as a lovely, fictional, warm world. I also grew to enjoy some of Doc Martin's rude mannerisms and even adopted a few of his milder behavioural traits (for example, saying, 'Stop speaking' to people who are wittering constantly in one ear while you are concentrating on performing a minor surgical procedure).

Several patients have been amused by my name over the years and many used to point out that their boots or shoes were named after me, but more recently they point out my connection with the TV series and ask if I have heard of it. I usually tell them that I'm the original or real Doc Martin and that I should get some recognition (financial, hopefully) from ITV. I am, of course, aware that there have been many, many GPs with the first name Martin before me, but I hope you will allow me my little indulgence. Several patients have also suggested that I should include their recent medical story if I did write to ITV, or, indeed, write about my experiences as a GP. Friends have said the same when I have shared some of the tales of the week's events at work – funny or sad, and suitably anonymised.

I realised, after nine years in medical school and in training posts, and then over thirty years as a GP, that I had seen and heard so much of what could be of interest to other people that I should write some things down and share them. Fortunately, I have kept some work diaries and, in other cases, recounted events often enough to still remember them clearly. I also have a bundle of to-and-from airmail letters from my brief time working in Africa, which my mum had kept safe, and secret, for thirty years.

Another title I considered for this medical memoir was *Adam Kay Ruined My Life*. The main reason should be apparent to any one of the millions who've read his first book, in particular. It is a really funny, thoughtful and moving memoir of his days in hospital training roles, mostly in the Obstetrics and Gynaecology speciality. I cannot attempt to compete with that book and I also have to point out that at least one of his anecdotes is remarkably similar to one of mine featured in this book. My anecdote is also true, as my family and friends will attest to, as I have been telling it, and many of the others here, for many years. Apart from Dr Kay, there are several other famous writers who qualified in medicine in the UK and practised for a while before leaving the NHS to become full-time writers (I am thinking particularly of Jed Mercurio and Michael Mosley). I have no pretensions of having their great writing skills, but I was hoping that my more extended career may have given me the chance of more exposure to a different variety of medical situations.

Before I become too smug or self-righteous on this matter, however, I recently read a news report of another local GP who has just retired at age seventy-nine, who plans to write a memoir. Absolute credit to him for working in the NHS for so long. I feel genuinely humbled.

The main thread of the book is about the day-to-day experience of becoming firstly a doctor and then a GP. It is not intended to be a specifically personal memoir based on extracts from my personal diary. It is also not bursting with too many bloody or gruesome stories that you might expect in *Casualty*, apart from the stories from when I was actually working in Casualty. It is based on me looking out at the world from within the NHS, rather than back at myself, although, admittedly, my interpretation of NHS structures is of course subjective, personal and a bit tongue-in-cheek; in summary, this is not a textbook.

I hope there is enough of training, hospital and General Practice experience present in these pages to entertain, amuse and maybe even inform you a bit.

I hope you enjoy it.

My Home Visit

I was four years old and living with my family in Salford. I had been ill, in bed, with a respiratory infection and fever. Our family GP, Dr Agarwal, visited our house and came upstairs to see me. He was calm, kind and authoritative. He opened his case and took out a stethoscope and listened to my chest. I remember the stethoscope as being cold. I remember him scribbling on some paper and handing it to my mum. I remember her thanking the doctor, and her asking me to do the same, before he left. I remember sneaking out of bed to peer through the window at the doctor's posh car; we didn't have a car yet, nor did most of our neighbours. I sensed that this added to his importance.

From that time on, I told everybody that I wanted to be an 'Indian doctor'.

My only other childhood experiences of the medical profession were confined to regular attendances at the local hospital's Accident and Emergency department (A&E) because of concussion, or stitches for injuries sustained in the school playground or local park. With the exception of these usually minor scrapes, I was fortunate to enjoy a happy childhood. I lived with both parents and my older sister in a small semi-detached house on a, seemingly, perfect road to grow up on.

Dad was an electrical engineer, having gained his professional qualifications at night school, on the nights he wasn't collecting door-to-door insurance. Prior to that he had some exposure to electrical work while doing his national service in the Royal Corps of Signals. He had been based in the Far East, spending a year in Hong Kong and then Singapore. He had narrowly avoided being sent to war in Korea and he led us to believe that his placements were therefore relatively cushy. His most dangerous exposure during his service was to a fire in the Hong Kong military telephone exchange, which he had apparently (accidentally) caused.

Mum had a longer CV, which included secretary, cinema usherette, pub and golf-club barmaid, auxiliary nurse, community audiologist and finally, local government officer (LGO) in a hospital A&E department. Fortunately, this last post was both after my spell of frequent accidents and also at a different hospital to the one I attended about them.

At one end of our road sat our junior school; the school had a large playing field and even its own indoor swimming pool, built by the parents' association. I mean, literally; built by volunteer parents under the supervision of a local builder who also had children at the school. At the other end of the road was a lovely park. This had a playground, playing fields, cafe, putting green, duck pond, tennis courts, bandstand, trees. My friends and I spent most of our childhood, outside school time, playing there; shouted home for our teas before running back there. Also on the road was a selection of shops, including a chip shop, newsagents, butchers, greengrocers, barbers, chemist. It was a nice little world.

Other early childhood time was spent helping out at my dad's allotment, playing with Lego, playing with Timpo toy soldiers, watching *Thunderbirds*, and reading *Famous Five* books. We liked cycling, often a lot further than my parents were aware. I also joined a nearby Sea Cadets unit with my friend, Peter. The cadet unit gave us great opportunities for outdoor stuff including rowing, canoeing, camping and hiking. We also had several longer trips to naval bases at Portsmouth and Lossiemouth airbases: trusted to travel there on our own, age thirteen, clutching our free train passes. For a few years I hoped that I might be able to look at a career in the Royal Navy, until I found out that I was far too short-sighted to be allowed to actually be based on a ship. I would have been able, at that time, to work in a shore-based role, but I really didn't see the point of that, so ruled it out.

The first time I remember actually considering medicine as a career was when I was sixteen, and on an exchange trip to Lünen, Salford's twin town in Germany. At that time, I had already selected my A-level subjects for when I went back to school after the holidays. I was vaguely thinking of a career in engineering, but was also planning on continuing learning German in the hope that I might get to study in Germany too, for a year at least. In the university curriculum (UCCA) book, there were photographs of some spectacular civil engineering projects abroad and I thought that this looked like an exciting career. It may well have been, but my eyes were opened to the idea of a medical career by one of the other exchange-trip travellers, Craig.*

Craig was twenty years old so was a few years older than the rest of us on the trip. He had just finished his second year as a medical student, and entertained us all with amusing and interesting tales about his studies so far. It all seemed a bit more intriguing than my previous career ideas, based as they were on a few photographs in the UCCA book. I asked Craig about the qualifications needed to get into medical school and about the work needed once there. He thought that good A-level grades were needed but that being a doctor was not inherently academi-cally challenging – just required a lot of studying and hard work.

Back at school, I went to see the headmaster and asked to change two of my A-level subjects to Physics and Chemistry,

---

* I recently found out that Craig was more exceptionally qualified to promote a career in the NHS than I realised then, as his mother was, officially, the very first patient to be treated by the NHS on 5th July 1948.

which were better suited to securing a place at medical school. He accepted this change after a month's delay to make sure that I would not change my mind again. In due course I applied for five different medical schools and received only one positive reply: this was from Manchester Medical School.

A Catholic Education

I had been lucky enough to attend a good secondary school, which also had an attached sixth form. The school itself was a direct-grant, Catholic, boys' grammar school run by the Christian Brothers – a religious order dedicated to teaching. Most of our teachers were members of this order and most of them wore their monklike habits while teaching. Like most of the other pupils, I had passed an entrance exam to get in, age eleven. My chances of attending a non-religious grammar school had been scuppered by the abolition of state grammar schools in our area. My primary school headmaster had then suggested to my parents that I should try the local Catholic grammar, which was still accessible; I was allowed to apply as my mum was Catholic, even though my dad was not, and we had not been church attendees. I understand that a few of the pupils were fee-paying, presumably if they had not passed the exam, but this was all kept a bit hush-hush.

The school had its own holy trinity: academic learning, Catholicism and rugby union. Such was the importance of rugby there that the first XV team rugby captain also automatically became The Head Boy. Several old boys had gone on to play for the English national team. My own rugby career was more extinguished than distinguished, and this was related in no small part to my extreme short-sightedness. Removing my glasses left me wandering around the pitch, wondering where the ball was and trying to decide if I should run towards or away from the blurred figures in the scrum, or maul or ruck, or line-out; whatever the hell was going on.

Other, later, ex-alumni included a guiding star of the Manchester Indie music scene and another is a current national union leader.

Discipline was strict at the school despite, or maybe because of, the religious and well-intentioned set-up through the Church. Corporal punishment was frequent and there was a permanent low-lying threat of sudden violence from the Brothers and also the few lay teachers. The deputy headmaster was also designated as 'The Punishment Master' and had a selection of canes with which to beat the most unruly of schoolboys. I was only a victim of this 'six of the best' punishment on one occasion, after answering back to a teacher about a piece of homework that I had submitted a day earlier, but the teacher thought that I hadn't done it and didn't appreciate me contradicting him. More common punishments included rapping knuckles with a ruler or being given 'the slipper', which meant being hit across the backside by a plimsoll rather than an actual slipper. Plimsolls were a light canvas and rubber sports shoe: the predecessor to trainers. Not as heavy, therefore, but it still hurt when you were whacked by a teacher, and the embarrassment of being bent over at the front of the class added to the punishment, of course.

I was also slapped across the face by Bro (brother) Victor, who was our religious teacher at the time. My sin had been not going to Mass on the preceding Sunday and then pretending I had.

Bro Victor, after walking around the classroom, then stopping in front of me, who he and the rest of the class knew to not be a proper Catholic – 'Did you go to Mass yesterday, boy?'

Eleven-year-old me, starting to blush – 'Err, yes.'

Bro Victor – 'Interesting. Mmm. What was the sermon about?'

Me, thinking the game was up but feeling like I had to try to keep up the pretence – 'Err. It was about God.'

Bro Victor – 'Go on.'

Me – 'And man.'

Bro Victor – 'Yes?'

Me – 'And we should all love each other?'

Silence.

Bro Victor, now smiling broadly and stepping closer; his smile now almost as broad as the grins of my classmates, who I could see in my peripheral vision – 'You didn't go, did you?'

Me, shaking my head, reluctantly – 'Err, no, sir.'

Smack!

I was as shocked by the noise as much as by the impact of his hand on my left cheek. I felt tears welling up.

Bro Victor – 'That's for not going to Mass.'

I nodded and swallowed.

Smack!

Again on my left cheek.

Bro Victor – 'And that's for lying about it.'

He stepped away back to the front of the class. I tried to avert my teary eyes from my classmates, but thankfully they appeared to be avoiding my gaze, perhaps too embarrassed to look at me.

I was not smacked again by Bro Victor, as I did start to go to church in my efforts to try to become a believer. I also asked my classmates about the sermons or lessons that had been given, if I had missed Mass again.

Bro Victor was not the only sadist at the school. It may not surprise any older readers that our main gym teacher also appeared to take a keen pleasure in punishing and embarrassing pupils, particularly when we had forgotten our gym kits. His preference was a cricket bat and for the pupil to bend over a gym vaulting box. He would taunt the pupils first by asking them to select the cricket stroke he was going to use on them (square cut, cover drive, etc.). Whichever stroke you picked would only lead him to ramp up the impending terror by chuckling and saying that that particular stroke was the worse, or his favourite. I only suffered from that punishment on one occasion. Other substitute gym teachers were less violent and stuck to the traditional punishment for pupils who had forgotten gym gear, which was making you hang (by the arms) from the wall bars as long as you could while the gym session continued.

At the time, no one questioned these punishments; nor did they consider that the treatments were wrong. I never told my parents and I don't think that I or my classmates were left with any permanent physical or mental harm from the systemic violence, but it seems incredible that this level of child cruelty was still legal and widespread in the 1980s. Perhaps the only lifelong mark on me is my mistrust of organised religions and their abuse of power. It also seems that my classmates and I appear to have been relatively spared from some of the more extreme horrors of school abuse; it has recently been revealed that many of the boys at my school were victims of sexual abuse in the 1960s, and that the perpetrator moved on to continue his crimes at other Catholic schools in the area.

As you will have gathered, it was quite a strict school and the majority of the pupils, including me, toed the line and did what we were told to do. In truth, I lacked the imagination to think there was any alternative to behaving and studying as expected, most of the time at least. In fairness, some of my classmates and I skived off ('played truant') and missed double-history lessons a few times in order to play snooker at Rileys in Manchester. I also missed school one morning to attend a record signing by Kate Bush at Manchester HMV; the album being *Never for Ever*. I took a few photos and received a chaste kiss on the cheek from Kate for my efforts: a good result!

My family were, indirectly, very supportive of my school-work, but did not really need to get heavily involved in my studies, as I was quite good at managing homework and my revision timetable independently.

As an example, my dad came home from the pub one night and said, 'Some of the blokes in the pub said that their kids are doing their A levels. Shouldn't you be doing yours soon?'

I replied, 'I'm halfway through the exams, Dad. I've got one tomorrow and the last two next week.'

'Oh. OK. Carry on then.'

I carried on, and managed to get the necessary A-level grades and was good to go. I was the first member of my family to go to university, so they seemed even more excited than I was.

The night before I was due to start, my dad looked flustered and cornered me in the hall, saying, 'Your mum wants me to talk to you about sex.'

'What do you want to know?' I bluffed, while also becoming embarrassed.

'Very good. Well, if your mum asks, just tell her we've had "The Talk".'

'OK. Will do.'

He seemed as relieved as I that we had, between us, success-fully conspired to avoid further mutual embarrassment.

My parents had obviously seen starting at university as some kind of border between childhood and adulthood. I don't remember having any such ideas, but I do remember having a recurrent dream in the weeks leading up to it. In the dream I was stood at the roadside looking at the aftermath of a gruesome car accident, with several bleeding victims lying on the road. Other witnesses looked at me and shouted at me to do something. I felt overwhelmed and woke up, sweating and anxious. After a few repeats of the dream, the accident victims also turned to me, imploring me to help, and I stood, fixed to the spot, before waking. The dreams felt real and stayed with me for a few hours each morning. I was filled with self-doubt and wondered if I would ever be able to hack it as a doctor.

Before starting medical school, the only really positive doctor role model I had was the fictional Hawkeye character from the US TV series *M*A*S*H*. Apart from Dr Agarwal, of course.

Medical School

On the first day of teaching, we attended a two-hour introductory lecture, the purpose of which was to give an overall idea of the type of teaching we were to expect: this included some very graphic photographs of road traffic victims and patients undergoing major surgery. Several students walked out of this lecture, and several of these left the course itself during that first week. I think that the shock effect of the lecture was done, at least partly, in order to give students some sense of reality of medical practice. It was probably a shame, because some of the students who walked out may have come round to accepting the potential horrors of medicine more easily if they had been more gradually exposed to them.

The next shock came the following day. We were to visit the pathology department for an introduction to the dissection room. We were ushered into a very large room with a low ceiling, where twenty embalmed cadavers (dead bodies) lay on metal trollies. Each group of ten medical students were allocated one of these bodies to dissect over the course of the following year. The room had the appearance of a sci-fi movie. The corpses were those of people who had, kindly, donated their bodies for medical research. Their families would not be able to bury their remains for at least another year. This likely delay was known to the donors when they completed the application process, often years in advance of their deaths: donation being a very altruistic act.

We were to spend about four hours a week in the dissection room over the next two years and I don't recall anybody ever being disrespectful to the bodies. Some of the medical students appeared naturally more skilled and careful than others when learning how to dissect: they tended to become even better as the rest of us were sidelined a bit so that the dissections looked neater and more helpful for the rest of us to understand the niceties of the revealed anatomy. Many of these, unsurprisingly, later became surgeons. For the less skilled of us, it was a bit like being left to one side at school sports while the better footballers or cricketers were selected to play.

The other surprise on entering the dissection room was a large notice on the wall stating that it was forbidden to eat while in the room. I believe that this instruction was made as a sign of respect for the dead. When we first saw this, the thought of anyone contemplating food or eating while in such a room was so ridiculous that we could not imagine any reason for this sign being needed. However, after a few months at medical school, and with the obvious increase in familiarity with the dissection room, students often started to talk about lunch towards the end of the two-hour dissection sessions. Everybody was still happy to comply with the rules, though, and wait till we got to the snack bar to eat.

The medical school also housed a pathology museum, which was a grand word for what was a single room containing large formalin-filled jars containing diseased organs and other body parts. The most disturbing of these contained the small, preserved grey bodies of newborn infants with severe genetic deformities. The museum was locked but available to enter for specific research purposes. It was a grim place even for those whose sensitivities had become reduced over time.

Digs

I was lucky enough to meet a group of fellow medics who had room for me in their digs, so I joined the other six in an old Victorian semi, with one shared bathroom and a run-down kitchen. The cellar was ideal for parties once we covered the walls with film and music posters. The house was tatty and overcrowded, especially when partners or friends stayed over: fourteen of us sharing the facilities was a bit of a stretch. Medics were inclined to hang around together because of their rotas and timetables. We generally had far more lectures and timetabled hours, but there was a tendency for medics to be viewed as snooty or having a superiority complex because they didn't always mix much.

The first party we had was on a Saturday night and was officially a birthday party for James, one of the fellow medics. We had bought plenty of alcohol and most guests turned up with more. At around 11 p.m., there was a lot of banging at the front door: loud and sustained enough for us to hear from a music-filled cellar. A few of us answered the door to three leather-and-denim-clad bikers at the door.

'We live next door and if you don't turn off that music we'll batter any blokes in there,' was their charming opening gambit.

One of the 'blokes' behind me muttered, quietly, that he was off to put on a dress, thankfully out of earshot of our neighbours.

I replied to them, 'I'm really sorry, but we've only got speakers in the cellar. We didn't think anybody could hear it.'

'Well, I live in the cellar next door and I can fuckin' hear it!' snorted one of the bikers.

'We had no idea, sorry. I'll go and tell James to turn it down. It's his birthday.'

The magic word, birthday, appeared to have a great effect on the attitude of the cellar-dweller. 'Oh, sorry. We didn't know it was a birthday. We just thought it was going be every fuckin' weekend, 'cos you're students.'

'No, it's a birthday,' I said. 'It won't be every weekend, but we'll turn it down anyway.'

'It's OK, we didn't know it was a birthday. Carry on.'

James was stood next to me by then. He had been uncharacteristically quiet, especially for a rugby player, and especially as he was not completely sober.

He spoke, 'Why don't you guys come in; you're very welcome.'

The bikers looked at each other, nodded, then walked straight in and down the steps to the cellar. They stood out a bit from the pastel-coloured students there but were well behaved and left when the beer ran out, leaving the rest of us to finish the remnants of the wine and liqueur bottles. They were on nodding terms with us from then on and also came to a few more parties, at which they volunteered as, and acted as, bouncers.

This same house was used by a rotating group of us for the next five years, providing a base and a great social hub. Two of the housemates, John and Greta, were particularly social animals and arranged parties and trips out for us all: tennis matches, picnics, crown green bowling, theatre and hiking trips. It was like being in an old people's home for young fogies. It was a fabulous, secure home-from-home, that enabled us to study and work, increasingly hard during our years at university.

Community: Medicine

With the exception of Statistics, the Community Medicine (CM) lectures were the least well-attended lectures in the pre-clinical years at medical school, especially among the students who planned to become surgeons, who had little interest when there was no anatomy. Community medicine, or public health as we call it today, was interesting for those of us who were leaning towards a career in General Practice. Plus we got to go on a few trips out with our tutor. I suspect the trips were not selected for their educational value but because they showed the more unusual aspects of the team's work: more entertaining than most of the day-to-day stuff.

The most anticipated of these trips was the visit to the local ladies' prison, in order to see the type of health services on offer for the inmates. This was fascinating. Who wouldn't want to visit a prison, as long as you can get out at night?

The prison smelt of carbolic and cabbage. Our tutor led four of us through security and into the medical clinic and sickbay area, in order to show us the type of services offered. We were more fascinated with, and keen to catch a glimpse of, the unfortunate inmates, although equally keen not to be spotted staring at them, in case any took rightful offence. In reality, of course, we stood out as far more uncomfortable and incongruous in that setting than any of the prisoners and had a few insults and comments shouted or muttered at us as we shuffled nervously through. The prison was cold, bleak and sad, and felt more so as we exited into the car park and that lovely spring day, a few hours later.

Another entertaining visit was to one of the Manchester Airport airline food-preparation kitchens. The local community health unit had some responsibility for checking that food safety regulations were being properly followed, as food poisoning was potentially more troubling and serious at 30,000 feet, especially for the pilot and co-pilot, who were not allowed to eat the same dishes in case of contamination. The kitchens were in a massive warehouse near to Wythenshawe. We were shown around the food preparation areas for the Economy cabins first, before moving up through Business and then First classes. The ultimate quality level was the amazing food that was intended for the Concorde passengers, together with all the proffered silverware, crockery and crystal wine glasses. Sadly, we did not get to taste even the Economy grub and settled for a meat pie when we got back to medical school.

They were quite keen on projects in CM. The first I undertook was a study of a local family's interaction with health services, which meant looking at and cataloguing how hard life was for families with handicapped (the terminology of the time) children. I interviewed a lady in her flat, a single parent who lived with her two children halfway up the tower block. The lifts were not working on the day I visited: apparently a frequent problem. Her small children both had Down's syndrome and both suffered from other serious heart conditions. Their overall developmental problems were at the more severe end of the Down's spectrum and they were likely to need a lot of support throughout their lives. At that age they appeared to spend most of their time engaging with hospitals for outpatient appointments, followed up by admissions for surgery. The flat was tiny and overcrowded, and every room was filled with washing, drying on wooden maidens.

'They both still have a bit of a problem keeping dry at night,' their mum said when she noticed me looking at all the wet clothes. Followed up with, 'And in the daytime, too.'

As well as telling me about the children, she told me about herself, including her perception and experience of medical mishaps and also her separation and divorce. Her life was tough.

Their lives were tough.

Really tough.

I left the flat with my notes, ready for my project. Even then I realised that the project itself was a side issue and that the real aim was to expose students like me to the hardships suffered by so many but to whom we would likely have had no previous exposure. I would like to think that I already had some empathy for people whose lives were a struggle, but I am sure that this visit also added a little to my understanding. I continue to have respect for families and patients for whom life's struggles are so difficult and yet easily forgotten by the rest of us. For many of us, bad things rarely happen and when they do, they pass quickly with no permanent consequences. For carers, every day can be a struggle, even when the burden is accepted freely because of parental love.

My second project was looking at the provision of cervical screening in the Manchester area: mostly focusing on how to increase uptake of the service in those patients who were at highest risk. I also conducted a review into the search for the cause of cervical cancer. At that time, it was being postulated that human papillomavirus (HPV) may be the cause, although other viruses were also in the frame as potential causes. Fast forward to today: HPV is the proven major cause, for which there is now an effective vaccination, which is proving so successful that the hope now is that cervical cancer may be eliminated completely in the UK. This is a huge breakthrough. There have been many amazing developments and improvements in medicine during my career, but rarely is there one that has transformed patients' future health prospects so fundamentally.

Ward Rounds

It's only in your third year as a medical student that you begin to think of yourself as a proper medical student: halfway to being a doctor. It was in our third that we began to visit hospitals and meet patients and wear our white lab coats in public.

During the summer holiday before, I was lucky enough to shadow an A&E senior registrar, Dr Andy Redwood, who my mother knew, having recently retired from the same department. Dr Redwood was an enthusiastic teacher who taught me how to suture properly, a skill I was able to use confidently throughout my career. Dr Redwood became a stalwart of A&E and emergency medicine: working and teaching for many years, going on to national and international renown in these fields.

Term started and I was sent to study and work in a nearby teaching hospital. On our first day, we were each allocated a named hospital inpatient to interview, in order to then 'present' their case to the group and tutor at a later teaching session. I went to the designated bed, but the patient wasn't there. I walked to the ward office, knocked and went inside. The four nurses there glanced up and then quickly looked away when they realised I was only a medical student, the lowest of the low in the hospital pecking order. My face reddened with awkward embarrassment.

'Excuse me,' I said. 'Please can I ask where Mr Beckinsale is?'

Nothing.

I understood. They were busy, and I was a nuisance. I walked further into the office and approached a nurse who was sat near to the notes trolley. She sighed and looked up.

I tried again. 'Sorry to bother you. Please can you tell me where Mr Beckinsale is? I've got to speak to him.'

She looked at me and said, 'He's gone for an ERCP.'*

'Oh, OK, thanks. What's an ERCP?' I asked.

'What's an ERCP?' she said, this time more loudly and directed to the room, generally.

This prompted gales of laughter from the other nurses.

Then to me, still loudly, 'You're a medical student and you don't know what an ERCP is?'

'No. Sorry. What is it?' I said, having little dignity left to lose.

The nurses stared at me, all smiling and enjoying the sport of humiliating a gormless med student.

She paused and also blushed a little. 'It's an investigation.'

The nurses went back to reading and writing their reports.

'Thank you. What does it stand for?' I asked, with my pen poised over my notebook.

'It's a test. You'll have to look it up; we're busy. Shut the door on your way out.'

The following day I returned to interview Mr Beckinsale, who was happy to talk to me and to share the story of his illness. None of my fellow students had heard of an ERCP either when I presented the case to them and our tutor.

Later that year, I was attached to a general surgical unit at Manchester Royal Hospital. While there, students were expected to interview one of the ward patients and present their case to the other students on the ward round. This was often quite intimidating, as the ward round was also attended by a professor, other doctors, the ward sister, several nurses, a pharmacist and a physiotherapist. All of these people were usually stood around the notes trolley as it was wheeled up and down the ward, with

---

* Endoscopic regrograde cholangiopancreatograph. No wonder she didn't attempt that. This is a procedure combining an upper gastro-intestinal endoscopy (gastroscopy) with X-rays, done in order to help diagnose and treat problems of the bile and pancreatic ducts.

the more senior doctors and nurses nearest the trolley, and the students a few rows away, at the back.

I had been called through to the front to present my patient to the assembled team. The case, as I saw it, was fairly straightforward and I was able to answer the questions put to me by the surgical professor, and also the more targeted questioning from the senior registrar, who was keen to establish the hierarchy on the ward.

Relieved, I slunk back to my place at the back.

James, a fellow student, was up next. He presented the medical history of his patient, a lady of eighty-four, who was due to have a bowel operation the next day.

'You say that this lady has a pacemaker?' said the registrar.

'Yes,' said James.

'When was it fitted?'

'Six months ago,' he replied.

'And do you know how long the pacemaker battery will last?'

'Ten years,' replied James, quietly confident that he knew the history well enough to avoid the usual planned public humiliation that the registrar was trying to achieve.

The professor seemed to wake up at this point and decided to join in again. He smiled over his half-moon glasses. 'And who wants to live to ninety-four?' He smiled again, soaking up the grins of the assembled crowd, and also amused at his own wit.

'Someone who's ninety-three, sir,' said James.

'Err, quite,' said the professor, smile now gone. 'Next patient, please, sister.'

One—nil to James, who grinned at me.

We had escaped the ritual humiliation of the ward round, for now, at least.

* * *

One of our biggest challenges was getting to lectures and hospitals, as only one of our tutorial group had a car. Bus services to the university were good, but not to the other outlying hospitals, so we cycled to many of them. This led to some problems turning up with all of the standard medical student equipment: stethoscope, auroscope, ophthalmoscope, tendon hammer,* BNF,† tape measure. We had been asked not to attend clinics with any bags as these looked unprofessional. One particular orthopaedic surgeon was wise to us turning up, just on time, on our bikes.

'Can I borrow your stethoscope, please?' he asked me, in front of a patient who had a painful knee.

'Sorry, Mr Babel, I don't have it with me today,' I said.

'Oh!' he said, stepping back in mock surprise. 'In that case I will borrow your BNF, then.'

'Sorry, Mr Babel, I don't have that with me, either, today.'

'Oh! In that case I will borrow your auroscope, as I want to check this poor gentleman's ears.'

'Sorry, Mr Babel, I don't have that, either, today.'

Mr Babel, now to the patient: 'Your life in their hands, eh? What do you think of that, Mr Diggle?'

At the end of the clinic, Mr Babel spoke to us in a more conciliatory tone. 'You might think I'm being mean to you, but it's very important to be completely professional in front of patients. It wouldn't do for me to turn up in the operating theatre, having left my scalpel at home, would it?'

None of us answered his rhetorical question.

'I asked you all a question,' he said.

Oops, not rhetorical, after all.

'No, sir,' we replied together, like naughty schoolchildren.

'I hope you've all learnt a valuable lesson today.'

---

* This is a small rubber-ended instrument used to test reflexes, often seen on television when doctors use it to hit patients just below their knees.
† *British National Formulary* – this is the standard pharmaceutical reference book in the UK. It is the bible for prescribing.

The chief lesson we learnt was that we should try to buy a car as soon as possible, which in my case was in the week after qualifying. Our morning of humiliation at his hands was completed as we cycled out of the hospital on our way to another; he drove his powder-blue Mercedes through a large, muddy puddle, splashing John and Greta. They were convinced that he had done it on purpose and were equally convinced they had seen him in his mirror, laughing.

The infectious diseases hospital was where we expected to learn about exotic and tropical diseases. Surprisingly, though, many of the most ill patients there were suffering from severe manifestations of more mundane, domestic infections such as chicken pox, and we saw another with late brain complications of measles. Another, a child, was ill with tetanus. All of these are often assumed to be trivial illnesses or beaten by vaccinations but, as we then learnt, they are only just beneath the surface, waiting to pounce if our guard is dropped.

One of infectious disease consultants spoke to us about the prevention of gastrointestinal infections while abroad and described a Nile cruise that he and his wife had recently been on. They had been the only two holidaymakers on that trip who hadn't succumbed to Pharaoh's Revenge, as he called it, so were suspected of having a secret preventative antibiotic regime by the other travellers. The real secret, he claimed to us, was that he and his wife had drunk a neat whisky before meals, without ice. He believed that the alcohol was itself antimicrobial.

Please join the queue, behind me, for funding into further research of this theory: perhaps a double-blind-drunk trial.*

---

* A double-blind trial is one in which the participants and investigators are initially excluded from, or 'blind' to, the knowledge of which drug/treatment the patient is receiving.

It's a Fair Cop

I was staying at my parents' house, in Salford, for the weekend. On the Saturday night, my dad allowed me to borrow the family Vauxhall Viva estate so I could drive to a friend's party in Sale, south of Manchester. I was well-behaved and made one pint of lager last throughout the whole evening, and I left the party at 1 a.m. I was turning onto the main road when a policeman, on foot, waved to me to pull over. I did this, nervous because of the smell of beer on my breath and wondering what I had done. He took his helmet off and climbed into the front passenger seat.

'Can you take me to Moss Side centre?' he asked, while effectively commandeering the car. 'It's all kicking off.'

'Err, yes, of course,' I said, relieved that I was not in any kind of trouble.

Moss Side was about four miles away. We set off and tootled along at thirty miles an hour.

After a few moments I thought I'd better ask him, and did.

'Err, can I speed?'

He looked a bit distracted, but turned towards me and said, 'Yeah, I suppose so. A bit.'

Not quite the ringing endorsement I had hoped for, which might have allowed me to floor the accelerator and enjoy full police protection while doing so. I therefore went about fifty miles an hour till we got near to Moss Side. He directed me to a community centre, where I could see several groups of men confronting each other.

The policeman told me to stop, thanked me and got out. He put his helmet back on, vaulted over a traffic barrier and set off running towards the melee. As far as I could see, he was on his own at that point, although I could hear a police siren getting closer.

Rather him than me, I thought to myself.

Year Four

We were now embarking on five different nine-week residential placements. Our first was at a children's hospital. The staff there treated medical students far more respectfully than we had come across in the adult hospitals. There was also a mixture of cheeriness and optimism that sat alongside the gloomy feel on the wards full of children with serious, potentially life-threatening, illnesses. This was forty years ago and thankfully, many or perhaps most of those diseases now have a much higher likelihood of survival.

Much of our time there was spent in observing rather than hands-on practice. When on call we saw acutely ill children admitted from home or transferred from a local A&E and were able to take a history and commence initial investigations, but we always had close support from the junior doctors on site.

Additional work while there included undertaking a written paediatric project, which involved quite a lot of research, alongside suggestions from our clinical tutors. My project involved looking at the differences between using tubes inserted in the veins or arteries of neonates'* umbilical cords to administer drug treatments or transfusions. My role was really just to trawl through published trials and articles to try to confirm the risk-versus-benefit ratio of these procedures, concluding with suggestions on minimising the risks.

The next two placements, in medicine and general surgery, were spent at another teaching hospital. Here, we were expected to take far more of a role in admitting and caring for patients, often

---

* Babies aged four weeks and under.

shadowing and assisting junior doctors. This included on-call at nights and weekends, which was a big shock to the system. On the surgical team, we were also able to spend a lot of time observing, and then assisting, the surgeons in the operating theatre.

Assisting surgeons in theatre was intimidating at first, partly because of the work of holding retractors and passing instruments to the surgeon, but also because of the questions asked of us by the surgeons or their registrars. Many of them were reasonable with their attitudes and questions, but a significant minority took every opportunity to try to humiliate students, making them the butt or punchline of every joke. It was clearly a rite of passage for the student and a perk for the nastier surgeons. The questions themselves were often reasonable ones about anatomy, but even correct answers were turned back on the student with sarcasm so that the theatre staff could have a giggle. Students were usually addressed as 'you' or, in my case, 'hey you, the fourth year with glasses on', rather than by name.

I suspect that the whole thing may have felt even more intimidating for the female students or those with overseas origins, although overt sexism and racism were not apparent; there were plenty of female and ethnic minority students and doctors in hospitals at that time. In particular, there was a cohort of intimidatingly efficient female junior doctors in that hospital already, a few years older than us, and already breaking down barriers.

Despite this culture of low-level bullying, the overall experience was incredibly exhilarating and, at last, it felt that this was what we had trained for. The junior doctors were also helpful and appreciative of any practical help we offered, giving them a chance for a well-needed food or toilet break on their otherwise relentless shifts. In addition, we got the chance to see patients in outpatient departments and then present them to the consultants, as well as sitting in on some of their consultations.

'It Got Lost'

During the nine-week surgical student placement, I spent a few days shadowing the surgical registrar, Neil, which meant I followed him around and sat in on clinics as well as being able to assist during a few operations. One morning, Neil was bleeped by an A&E doctor with a referral. We went down to see the patient as soon as the clinic finished.

The patient was somebody who worked at the hospital. He had managed to get a shampoo bottle (Vosene) lodged in his rectum. He claimed that he had slipped and fallen onto this while in his bathroom. He had tried to remove it, but his anal sphincter muscles were now in spasm and had effectively pushed it higher up. He must have been in a great deal of discomfort in order to overcome the extreme embarrassment of turning up at hospital, especially the one he worked at. The discomfort and embarrassment were to get a bit worse during and after the examinations by the registrar and then myself. We became aware of a buzzing sound when we examined his abdomen, and then even more so when doing a rectal examination. The noise was coming from somewhere inside his abdomen. This was confirmed by listening with a stethoscope.

At that point, the patient said, 'There might be something else up there, too.'

'What do you mean?' asked Neil.

'Err, I was just trying one of these vibrator thingies and it got lost,' replied the patient.

'What about the shampoo bottle, then?' asked Neil.

'I used that to try to get the vibrator out, then that disappeared, too. Can't you just get them out now?' the patient responded.

'No chance, especially as there is another foreign body in there. We might need to arrange a procedure under general anaesthetic,' said Neil.

The patient looked even more uncomfortable, in every sense, if that was even possible. The next step was to arrange an X-ray to confirm how far the vibrator had migrated up this chap's colon: not too far, thankfully. It was quite a shock to see such a startlingly clear X-ray image of the device in his abdomen, complete with two batteries. Neil wondered whether they might be Duracell batteries and give the chap a period of more extended discomfort during his wait for surgery. In the end, he had to wait overnight until a colonoscopy could be arranged the next morning. I was not able to attend for this as I was in another theatre with the consultant, but Neil was keen to tell me afterwards that the procedure had gone well and that the vibrator was still humming on its removal.

I think most hospital staff are aware of similar cases turning up in their A&E departments and the stories may well become embellished a little on retelling. If you have heard any of these then you may think they are urban myths. I suppose some might be. This one is true.

God Only Knows

Next up for us was a large psychiatric unit in another hospital, and this provided the opportunity to interview and present cases in outpatient clinics and during inpatient ward rounds. The pace of events was generally much slower than during our previous placements, although this became more hectic and frantic when we were observing and also helping during out-of-hours sessions, which was when most of the acutely ill and psychotic patients presented. We were often involved in helping to manage patients while they were at their most distressed and disturbed, and at highest risk to themselves and others. At first it was a shock to see some patients at the extremity of their illnesses, many with violent verbal and physical outbursts. Some of these required physical restraint by three or four nurses, plus available students, sometimes holding the patient down and giving them sedative injections. This kind of scenario was uncommon and unpleasant, but sometimes necessary.

Most of the inpatients had initially been admitted under 'sections', which referred to different sections of The Mental Health Act, allowing initial admission and treatment against the patient's will, if necessary. Patients were regularly reviewed and their rights protected by the acts until they were well enough to make their own decisions.

Some patients were less dramatic but equally disturbing. One such chap was obviously an intelligent man, although he was quite intense during general conversation. After a few minutes of talking, it became clear that he had a fairly high opinion of himself and was looking down upon the rest of us. Further questioning revealed why: he was absolutely convinced that he was God, and this belief was totally unshakeable. Sadly, we moved on to another hospital before finding out how He progressed.

Obstetrics

The last of our fourth-year placements was at an Obstetrics and Gynaecology department. I was placed with Mr Stephens' team. The same medical staff worked in both units. On the gynaecology side of things, we were expected to help with the admission of patients for routine operations and for emergencies, in addition to attending clinics and assisting in theatre. There, we even had the opportunity to undertake some more minor procedures, while under supervision. The consultants and registrars seemed a lot less confrontational and more helpful than the general surgeons had been. We were also included in the formal out-of-hours duty rotas and were expected to be there alongside the medical staff, for much longer and busier shifts than we had previously been expected to do. Most of the out-of-hours time was spent dealing with obstetric cases, often culminating on the labour ward.

For completion of our training we were required to attend and assist at a certain number of 'normal' deliveries, as well as more problem cases. Many of those ended with instrumental delivery if the babies showed signs of distress or prolonged delay. Instrumental delivery could be by ventouse* or by forceps or even caesarean section, at which medical students were frequently asked to assist. We mostly assisted Mr Stephens, but also, quite often, Mr Farookh, the Egyptian senior registrar. He was friendly and helpful, but also had a bit of a reputation as a ladies' man.

---

* Ventouse extraction involves a small vacuum cup attached to a chain, which is applied to a baby's head. This allows the safe use of a certain amount of force to try to help pull a stubborn term baby out if needed.

A reputation he was happy to cultivate, while wearing sunglasses and chain-smoking in the canteen.

'You see, I have to get the most out of this country before I go home,' he said. 'I like ladies. I like a nice drink. I like to smoke. Things will be different at home. I will be expected to marry a plain woman.'

Things were slightly different for him at Ramadan, too. This was in July, so there was an awful lot of daylight for him to cope with, and work around. We saw quite a lot of him, as we were usually on the same duty rotas. After sunset at around half nine, and work permitting, he would smoke five or six cigarettes before tucking into his tea. He would usually manage another meal before going to bed at midnight. He set his alarm for 4 a.m. and managed another half-packet of cigarettes and breakfast before either joining us or going back to bed if the labour wards were quiet. Things were much tougher during the daytime for him, as he strictly avoided any food or drinks or cigarettes, but worked as hard as anybody else without ever complaining.

The consultant, Mr Stephens, was an entertaining and charismatic fellow who drove a spectacular Jaguar sports car and wore colourful suits, garnished with a fresh carnation in the buttonhole. He had a charming bedside manner, making him popular with all of his patients, particularly the older gynaecology ones.

One day, in clinic, he was changing a lady's ring pessary.* He spoke to her conspiratorially. 'Do you know what you should do if this falls out in the supermarket, Ada?'

She shook her head. 'No, Mr Stephens.'

'Just kick it under somebody else. Then give my secretary a ring. I'll fit a bigger one.'

---

* A small plastic or rubber ring inserted into a patient's vagina, used to hold a prolapse in place, as an alternative to surgery: usually used if a patient was unsuitable for surgery.

Ada howled with laughter.

He was equally entertaining in theatre. I was assisting him with a particularly bloody and messy gynaecological operation, when he looked up at me over his half-moon spectacles. 'Does this put you off women? All this mess?'

I was not really sure how to answer this, especially in front of all the other doctors and nurses and theatre staff.

I muttered, 'Not really.'

'Well, it puts me off. Till I think of the alternative.'

On another occasion, he was being teased about his car by one of the theatre nurses.

She said, 'I need to get a new wheel for my Mini. I saw your flash car parked outside on my way in this morning and I thought that my whole car probably costs less than one of your wheels!'

'One of my wheels? I think it's worth less than one of my tyres. Cheeky bugger.'

Everyone in the theatre laughed. Nobody appeared to resent his wealth, or fancy lifestyle, and were always keen to ask him about where he had been over the previous weekend: usually at a horse or car-race meeting, unless he had been on-call, of course.

One morning during the ante-natal clinic, Mr Stephens asked me to run an errand to another hospital, in order to pick up some paperwork he had left there. 'Will you nip up to The Royal for me, to get those notes, at lunchtime?'

I answered, 'Of course, but I might have to leave now so that I can back in time for theatre.'

'Why, are you walking?' he said, grinning.

'No, sir, I've got a bike,' I replied.

'You can take my car,' he said.

'Really? I've never driven an automatic before.' Nor had I driven a Jag, or any sports car, or any other car with a 5.3 litre engine.

'It's just like a bumper car,' he said, and then added, 'But don't actually bump it. You can give it a bit of a whizz. You can normally get past a ton if you go on the motorway.'

He gave me the keys at the end of clinic, and I nipped to The Royal and back on the motorway. It was a beautiful car, but I did not even try to get up to 'a ton' as I was petrified of having an accident or getting a speeding ticket. It was probably the nicest car I have ever driven in my life.

Mr Stephens called me to his office on my last day at his unit: also my last day in the fourth year. I went in. He was sitting behind his desk. 'When are you going on your elective?'

I replied, 'In three days, sir.'

'Somewhere in Africa, wasn't it?'

'Yes. Botswana,' I said.

'How are you funding that?' he asked.

'I've got a bank loan, sir.'

'Well, I'm sure you could do with a bit more. Take this.' With that, he handed me a cheque for £50.*

I was extremely surprised and equally grateful.

'What's this for? I can't take that; thank you anyway.'

He looked a bit embarrassed. 'It's for all the help you've given me. You've assisted me on quite a few private sections.'

'I have to assist anyway, whether it's private or not,' I said.

'No. Keep it. I get paid plenty and you've been really good. I hope you are thinking about doing Obs and Gynae as your career?'

'Well, I was planning on General Practice, but I've really enjoyed the placement here, so I'm not sure now,' I said.

'Good man,' he said, and stood up to shake my hand. Little wonder he was so popular with patients and staff.

---

* £50 in 1984 is worth about £205 today.

Botswana

Between our fourth and fifth years there was a three-month break during which we were expected to do an 'elective'. This was a period in which you 'elected' a work placement. Several students I knew had selected posts in specialities that they were considering for their careers, often in highly regarded hospitals and departments within the NHS. Many of us chose to work overseas. I had been looking enviously at a posting in rural Canada, which involved travelling to outlying clinics by seaplane! It turned out that this particular placement was, unsurprisingly, in such demand that it had been booked up many years earlier for the time I was free.

One of my friends had been accepted by two different hospitals in Africa: one in Kenya and one in Botswana. He chose to go to Kenya with another of our housemates and passed on the information about the Botswana placement to me. I wrote to the manager of the hospital and was accepted. Great news; I just needed to sort out the finances. The hospitals that accepted elective students tended to offer free accommodation and some food, so I just needed funds for the flights and some living costs for my time there. Flights were much more expensive in those days, so I needed to arrange a bank loan (the total flight costs in sterling are similar even now, some thirty-nine years later). My parents were helping me by supplementing my student grant at the time, but could not afford any extra. I arranged an appointment with my Barclays Bank manager. He listened to my plans and my request for a deferred bank loan, as I would not be able to start any repayments until I (hopefully) started working as a doctor the following August.

He looked a little bemused and said, 'I don't see why we should be funding your African holiday; it's too risky.'

I could not let my opportunity pass and so I booked an appointment at another bank, NatWest, who had a reputation for being student-friendly. They certainly were to me, and agreed on a loan provided I changed banks and also got my father to act as a guarantor. He was able to do this, thankfully.

The best flights I could book from Manchester were with a Portuguese airline, changing at Lisbon for an onward flight to Johannesburg. From there, I would fly with Air Botswana to the capital, Gaborone. I was to be picked up from there by somebody from the hospital I was going to work at.

I was dropped off at Manchester Airport by my parents, only to find my flight was delayed overnight as the Portuguese plane had burst a tyre on landing at Manchester. The other passengers and I were put up at an airport hotel overnight and flew out the next day. Unfortunately, there was no onward flight on that day, so I was put up in Lisbon for a further overnight stay and took off for South Africa two days later than originally planned. I was excited to be on the way properly, having only flown once before, on the exchange trip to Germany.

We landed for refuelling in Zaire (now the Democratic Republic of the Congo). I seemed to be the only passenger awake at the time. I was aware how dark it was on the ground, before and after refuelling, for many hours, with no visible house or street lights. We landed in Johannesburg just after dawn, so I tried to catch up on some sleep in the departure lounge before I caught my next plane to Gaborone, a short flight on a propeller plane. Gaborone airport was not much larger than a bus depot. There was nobody there to greet me, so I got a taxi to the *actual* bus rank, where hundreds of people were milling around the edge of a dusty, open space, with a dozen buses parked up in the middle.

An obvious tourist with my brand-new rucksack and duffle bag, I walked up to the bus bound for the village I was heading to. A young lad grabbed my bags from the ground and clambered up a ladder on the side of the bus. I wasn't sure if I was being robbed, and I was still a bit wary as I watched my bags being flung onto the top of the bus, and into a small roof rack.

'Are they safe up there?' I shouted.

'It's my job, mister,' he replied, irritated.

I stood with the crowd, waiting for the driver to let us on the bus. A few minutes later another, younger, lad approached me, directly. He was dragging a crate of oranges behind him.

'Ten thebe!' he announced to me. I was aware that this was a small amount of money, probably only a few pence. I was also aware that all eyes were upon me. I felt self-conscious and thought that I was expected to barter with him.

'Five thebe?' I countered, hopefully, trying to show off my negotiating skills.

'You cheat me, mister!' he responded and walked off, dragging the orange crate with him.

That had not gone well, to say the least; besides which, I really did fancy one of those oranges. I later found out that Botswana was one of the very few African countries in which bartering was not done and was regarded as an insult to the seller.

The bus door was soon opened and we were let on. I was told to sit near the back, as I would be one of the last passengers off. The bus was packed, with everybody else carrying their possessions, which soon filled the gangway. After five minutes we were on the open road, heading up past the large dam on the outskirts of town. I watched the shadow of the bus pass along the side of the road, and also the shadows of my bags on the roof, bouncing up and down as we hit every pothole. I was panicking in case one of them bounced up high enough to fall off. I was mentally rehearsing how I would shout out to stop the bus and try to get down the blocked passageway in order to go back and retrieve said bag from the road. Thankfully, this was not necessary and gradually the passengers thinned out as people got off at occasional informal stops on the road.

After a few hours, the remaining half-dozen passengers and I arrived at the village. We had stopped right by the hospital. My bags were thrown down to me by the bus driver's assistant, who still seemed bemused by me. I thanked him and stepped back from the road.

I had a quick look towards the village, which was made up of rondavelles – round, sandy-brown, single-storey huts with conical thatched roofs. Plumes of smoke came from each of these huts, leaving a strong smell of woodsmoke in the air. Underfoot was sand, apart from the narrow tarmac road. I waited for the bus to leave and crossed the road to the hospital, which was also single storey, with only a water tower and a small church tower rising above.

'Here at Last'

Through the gates into the hospital, I made my way to the office near the front entrance and introduced myself.

'Ah, you're here at last,' said the secretary.

I apologised for my unavoidable delay.

She told me that Dr Kirkby was giving a lecture and that I should follow her. She ushered me into the side of a classroom and I watched the last half-hour of a talk about antenatal care that he was giving to nurses and midwives.

After it finished, I met Dr Kirkby. He gave me a brief overview of my expected activities and then I was shown to my room in a small area off a corridor beyond the kitchen. The room was fairly spartan, with a bed, a desk, a sink and a metal wardrobe. I left my luggage there and returned to the hospital proper.

The other doctors were in clinic or theatre. Dr Kirkby asked me to go to the small morgue at the hospital and continue a post-mortem that had already been started; one of the other doctors would join me later. He warned me that the storage fridge was not working properly. I went to the small office-cum-morgue. I pulled the mortuary tray out of the broken fridge. The corpse was that of a child. That was a shock, to say the least. I had seen a few PMs but never for a child. I also had some experience with dissection, following the pathology training in the first two years, but again this was on the corpses of elderly people; never on children. The room was very hot and, unfortunately, things were a bit smelly. Somebody had already made the most of the expected incisions. I looked at the notes, which were on the desk in the room. It gave details of this poor child's illness, deterioration and death. It also looked like the PM had already been pretty much completed, apart from awaiting results from microbiology testing. I suspect I had been sent to the room just to occupy me until one of the other doctors was free. I did not have to wait long.

Dr Ian Baxter popped in. He told me that he had done the PM and now had the microbiology results. He asked me to check the brain cavity in the skull. The fluid there was cloudy and dull, whereas you would have expected it to be clear. I wondered if the child had died from meningitis. Ian confirmed this but pushed me a bit more to try to more specific. I was stuck. He told me that microscopy had confirmed that the child had died from cryptococcal meningitis. He had heard of this condition but never seen it before. I had never even heard of this, although I was vaguely aware that cryptococcus was an unusual type of fungus. He asked me to sew up the excisions and then to catch up with him on one of the wards. I sutured as asked, then tidied up and slid the drawer back into the fridge.

Today, I am aware that cryptococcal meningitis is associated with impaired immunity problems, especially with the human immunodeficiency virus (HIV) disease, and is often, nowadays, actually used as a marker of undiagnosed HIV in communities. Acquired immunodeficiency syndrome (AIDS) was initially first diagnosed in Botswana in 1985, but retrospective studies suggested that it was likely to have been already present in 1984. The causal virus later became officially known as HIV in 1986.

Botswana went on to experience one of the most severe HIV and AIDS epidemics in the world, developing the third highest national rates for a number of years. The current HIV prevalence in adults is around twenty per cent. I now believe that this poor child was an undiagnosed and very early victim of AIDS/HIV disease.

I met up with Ian again and he explained some more about the set-up at the hospital, and my small role in helping out. The hospital was a German religious mission hospital. Most of the staff were locals or Botswanan, at least. There were four doctors. Dr Kirkby was South African, originally an ENT specialist and also the clinical superintendent of the hospital, so spent a bit less time in clinical work than he had previously done. Dr Galtberg was a German paediatrician. Ian was Scottish, and was on a five-year voluntary placement via his Christian church. He was not a specialist and had completed his hospital GP training posts in the UK. He was there with his wife. The only other doctor there was another German, Dr Herman Weil, who was also a generalist. He, too, was accompanied by his wife and their two small children. All of the doctors had a broad range of skills, well beyond their usual roles in their home countries. The funding was, in those days, mostly from the Botswana government, but the doctors' wages and expensive equipment were provided by a German Lutheran mission. There were also several German nuns who were volunteering on the wards – all of them being trained nurses.

The hospital had four wards with around one hundred beds. There were two operating theatres and an X-ray room. I was expected to assist on the wards and in theatre, and to do outpatient clinics. I was also expected to be first on call on a one-in-two rota. This meant doing the usual five-day week and additionally being called first on every alternate night and weekend for emergencies on the wards or antenatal unit, or in the outpatient area. I would start this rota on the next day.

By now it was dark. I was so tired that I just climbed into bed, set my alarm for 6 a.m. and tried to catch up on some sleep. There was a lot of noise coming from the nearby village. It sounded like drums. It was all a little bit scary and added to my sense of being out of my comfort zone. I felt homesick, so got up, sat at the desk and wrote my first airmail letters home.

I tried again to sleep but couldn't due to the vast number of mosquitos dive-bombing me. I got up and swatted as many as I could, before I spotted the broken netting over the open window. I closed the window but still had a cloud of mosquitos to get through before I could get much peace. It was too hot to sleep under the blanket and poking my head out was a bit challenging, too. I eventually fell asleep and I was woken up in the early hours by a surprisingly noisy fight between a huge spider and a cockroach on the concrete floor. I left them to it.

Time for Work

Breakfast in the staff canteen consisted of lukewarm mealie-meal (maize) porridge and a cold fried egg on bread. We then went en masse to the small church in the hospital grounds. The hospital staff were all expected to attend church. The service was in Setswana (the main language in Botswana) and I tried to follow the service and hymns as best I could from the booklets left on the pews. After that it was on to work.

I was put in with Dr Weil in the small outpatients department while he saw patients. This department was a fairly new section at the front of the hospital with two consulting rooms and an outside roofed waiting area with no sides, which tried to offer some protection from the sun. Patients usually turned up without an appointment and waited to be seen. Dr Weil showed me the handheld records that patients were supposed to carry with them whenever they had any medical treatments. This was an A4 piece of card folded twice and popped in a plastic sleeve. Many of the patients had lost the sleeves and the notes were understandably very worn and tatty having been carried around in bags and back pockets for years. Many had lost their records altogether.

Herman showed me how to prescribe for the patients, who could then take the script to the hospital pharmacy for dispensing, for free. There was a fairly limited list of drugs available, mostly antibiotics and painkillers. Some of these were injectable items that the patient would then bring back to the clinic room to be administered.

We also had the help of an outpatient aide in each room. Their main role was to translate the patient's Setswana language into English, and vice versa. They also helped to provide a cultural link between the patient and doctor, although there was obviously still a potential for them to add their own agenda to the consultation.

It was also possible to do some blood and other pathology tests, but these had to be used more sparingly than in the UK, partly owing to cost, but also owing to other practical issues. Many of the patients had travelled a long way to the hospital, often many days' travel, and would not be able to wait around for results. Some of the microbiology tests were done by the doctors themselves. For example, any swabs for venereal diseases were taken by the doctor, and, later, me, and then put onto a slide with appropriate dyes and viewed on a microscope. This gave an immediate diagnosis and allowed for rapid treatment.

Many of the conditions that presented that morning were very similar to what you might expect in the UK, although there was probably a higher presentation of venereal infections and gynaecology problems.

We broke for lunch after a five-hour morning surgery. Lunch was the same every day: a scoopful of bogobe, some carrots or beetroot and a ladle of curry sauce. The bogobe was a savoury porridge made from sorghum flour. Every week or so there was a bonus beef chop added to each plate. Lunch was a chance to catch up with the doctors and see what was going on in the hospital.

It was decided that I should do the afternoon session in outpatients, this time consulting on my own, although Dr Weil was next door for help and advice if needed. I had done consultations before, during my training, but not with the aid of a translator, which added an extra dimension to things, as I also had to try to manage her, to some extent. I am sure she felt exactly the same way about me.

My first session began. Most of the presentations seemed fairly straightforward. What was more difficult was knowing how far to investigate many of the patients and where to refer anybody for treatments such as routine surgery. I spoke to Herman about some of these patients to ask for his guidance. Some of them needed referral to the Princess Marina Hospital: the country's main and only large hospital back down the road in Gaborone. I kept a list of the names and planned to handwrite referral letters after the clinic finished. The last patient that afternoon left just as the sun was starting to set.

The sun sets very quickly that near to the equator, so it was pitch-black by the time I finished the letters and made my way back to my room.

After a quick wash, I walked to the kitchens to see if there was any food. I turned on the bright fluorescent light to see and hear a sheening mass of cockroaches scuttle off into the dark underneath the counters. After a few seconds, they had all gone and it was quiet again. All a bit disconcerting to say the least, but I still had a quick look round to see if I could find any covered food. I couldn't, but I sat down at a metal table to see if anybody else turned up. I had been told that most of the temporary staff or volunteers hung around in this area out of hours. After a short wait, some of the German volunteers came in. One was a medical student and three others were nuns. The student had just finished his second year at university so was not allowed to conduct medical consultations nor give medical opinions, but was still able to help out generally and gain a lot of valuable experience. The group were speaking German but kindly switched to English while I was there, although I was able to practice my O-level German when they were around. On this occasion, they had all brought some food from their rooms and, once again, kindly, shared this with me. They also showed me where there was some bread kept away from insect attack, together with a jar of peanut butter for night-time snacks. They told me that there was a small general store nearby that was still open for an hour after dusk.

They recommended trying the fat cake if I was very hungry. I made a mental note.

One of the orderlies now came looking for me. The midwives had asked for me to go to the labour ward. I felt increasingly nervous as I followed the orderly. I had some recent experience in obstetric care, especially as my last nine-week medical school posting had been in Obs and Gynae. I had delivered a number of babies and witnessed many more but hadn't had to make decisions about problem labours. I was conscious that the midwives would have had vastly more experience than I had, but they had specific roles and so did I. I also had the backup of the second on-call doctor, of course, if needed. I was aware, too, that most women in Botswana would expect to have their babies at home and that generally, only the higher-risk labours were dealt with in hospital.

I met up with the senior midwife on duty and she took me to see a few of the ladies who were in labour on the unit. One of these seemed to be progressing a bit slowly in her labour and she was screaming.

A lot.

'Has she had any analgesia?' I asked, trying to focus on things in a sensible, stepwise fashion.

'Of course she has!' said the midwife before laughing. 'We are not savages.'

'What has she had?' I asked, trying to sound confident, like a proper doctor.

'Paracetamol. Two,' she told me.

OK, that had told me.

'Could we not step this up at all?' I tried.

She smiled and told me some home truths. 'You see, our ladies are much tougher than your ladies in Europe. They don't usually need any help and certainly don't need painkillers just to have a baby.'

OK. That was me told again. Throughout my training and subsequent professional career, I have always realised that it is generally a good idea to listen to the nurses, sisters, charge nurses and midwifes. They usually had more experience in their individual specialities than most junior doctors, let alone medical students like me. It is at the very least a good idea to explore what they think one should do, even if you feel differently. If nothing else, it gives a clearer position for any negotiation.

'What do you think we should do?' I asked.

'Nothing at the moment. I was just letting you know that we might need to call you during the night. Maybe you should stay awake?'

I was happy with the short-term aspect of her plan but thought that I should actually try to get some sleep as I had a full schedule on the following day. I was also tired. I went back to my room for an hour, swatting more mosquitos and writing a few more airmail letters home.

After that, I popped back to the labour ward to find that things were progressing well, so I went back to my room to try to get some rest. I slept badly again as I was half-expecting to be woken for the labour ward, while being eaten alive by the mosquitos.

I must have fallen asleep, as I was woken up by my morning alarm. I diverted to the labour ward on my way to the church service. Both of the ladies had safely delivered healthy babies with no special interventions required. Apart from the paracetamol, of course.

Cases

I was now able to help out by assisting in the operating theatres. The range of surgical procedures performed by the doctors was quite astounding. At one of my first morning theatre sessions, the doctor who I was helping performed a ventricular shunt procedure, a tubal-ligation sterilisation, a uterine dilatation and curettage (D&C), cervical cautery for genital warts, removal of two rotten teeth, cautery to verrucae, ear suction, removal of a foreign body from a child's nostril, skin grafting for burns and, finally, reduction and setting of a Colles wrist fracture. Astonishing.

Overall, the most common operation done there was the caesarean section and this was usually done as an emergency, and often at night. Also of note was the extreme heat in the theatres: usually over forty degrees Celsius and incredibly hot for the surgeons and nurses in their green theatre gowns, caps and masks. We all left the operating sessions dehydrated and drenched in sweat, as well as in the patients' blood and bodily fluids. Rehydration was via a ready supply of the hot Milo drink consumed in large quantities by all of the hospital staff. This was a sweet, milky chocolate and malt drink further enhanced, by most of them, with the addition of three or four spoons of sugar. Far too sweet and sickly for me at first, but I was soon drawn into the club, although I managed to resist the extra sugar.

I was able to do a few minor surgery sessions on my own, setting fractures, excision of small lumps, removal of embedded thorns from skin, and also removal of foreign bodies from noses and ears. A surprisingly large number of patients attended with large insects stuck in their ears, with the creatures often still alive and wriggling, even after a few days. Some of these patients had travelled for many of those days just to get relief from such a distressing problem.

There was a lot of TB in Botswana at that time and many of the male patients, in particular, had been admitted early on in their disease for drug therapy. Most of these patients then completed their treatment courses as outpatients. This was itself problematic, as traditional TB drug regimes at that time were often up to two years. It was difficult to keep an eye on these patients, as many of them lived a long way from the hospital; many worked away in mines in Botswana and South Africa. Dr Kirkby was keen to reduce this regime to six months to try to aid compliance and to enhance the successful completion of their therapy.

I was asked to do a small project, looking at data from the previous three years' TB patients. I was looking at figures on defaulters, cures, deaths and relapses. The data supported the belief that many patients dropped out of the longer two-year courses, but that their cure rate at two years would have been no better than after six months. This data supported the change to a six-month drug regime at the mission hospital, at least as a first-line plan.

The children's ward was livelier during the day than I had seen on NHS children's wards, because the children's mums often stayed at the hospital throughout their child's stay. The wards were quieter at night, though, because the mums slept on the bed with their child or on the floor under the bed, and were able to offer comfort and reassurance in this strange place.

One of the long-stay patients on this ward was a twelve-year-old lad who was suffering from bacterial endocarditis (infection of the heart valves) connected with rheumatic fever as a smaller child. He required long-term intravenous antibiotics but was, happily, well enough to be discharged before I finished there. On reading through his records, I was surprised to see a clinic letter from Dr Christiaan Barnard. Dr Barnard was the surgeon who performed the first ever human-to-human heart transplant and was famous at that time, becoming a jet-setting celebrity, meeting the Pope, and appearing on chat shows and in gossip columns. Away from the world of celebrity, he had continued to do cardiology and charity work, and had seen this lad at one of clinics for underprivileged children. He had considered doing valve-replacement surgery but decided it was not necessary.

Back in outpatients, I was getting a bit more familiar with the presentation of illnesses by patients. There were some cultural differences, both in the presentation of illness and expectations for treatment. They tended to be a bit more demonstrative of the levels of pain and distress they were suffering. Some of these behaviours may have been altered by having to impress the doctor. One particular patient pointed to every part of his body when I asked where his pain was. When I asked how severe the pain was, he started to scream and shout in Setswana as he touched every part of his body and limbs again, in order. The doctor in the next room popped his head through the doorway to check everything was OK. I nodded that it was. The patient had politely paused for a few moments then restarted his apparently agonising tour of his body. He then mimed vomiting and diarrhoea, followed by gripping his abdomen tightly and spasmodically. He then sat back in his chair.

The translator looked at me with a completely straight face and said, 'No bad pain anywhere.'

'Are you sure? He looked like he had bad pain to me.'

She looked at her watch and then at the clinic room clock.

'Maybe some pain,' she conceded reluctantly.

She then appeared to start translating what the man was trying to say and we eventually got through the consultation.

I also tried to speed up a little, as she was obviously worried about the time and also the vast number of patients we had yet to see that morning.

Road Accident

After yet another long, hot day in the outpatients department, a man ran up to the door, shouting in Setswana. Dr Weil and his clinic aide came in to see what all the noise was about. The translator told us that there had been a terrible accident just outside the village. A lorry, carrying some schoolchildren and their teachers, had overturned. Some of them had been killed, but many were injured and some were still in the wreckage. Many were walking to the hospital.

Ian appeared from theatre. He decided to head off to the truck with a few nurses and an ambulance driven by one of the hospital orderlies. The rest of us were to set up a triage in the waiting room near the hospital entrance. A temporary morgue was also set up. Six children had died in the crash. There were several seriously injured children, one with spinal injuries and others with severe abdominal injuries. There were many walking wounded and others, less mobile, who had had been picked up by villagers and carried to the hospital. Thanks to the triage assessment, we were able to deal with the most urgent needs in the appropriate order. Both of the theatres were used for urgent abdominal repairs and then limb repairs and fracture management. I spent most of the evening and night suturing wounds for people who could be managed with local rather than general anaesthetic. I spent several hours suturing a severe facial and scalp wound for a teacher, whose forehead had been effectively peeled back over half of his head by the crash.

He had been very patient, despite his injuries, waiting for us to deal with those even more urgent than him. Ideally, he should have been given a general anaesthetic and had his surgery in theatre, but these were both full at that time with patients who had potentially life-threatening injuries. I used a lot of local anaesthetic and numerous sutures and he spoke to me throughout the procedure. He told me that the truck was used as school transport and that the whole class of fifty-six pupils, plus six teachers, had been on a day trip to Gaborone museum. On the way back, and quite near to the village, the truck had apparently burst a tyre and then hit a ditch, turning the truck over. He thanked me when I finished.

I was called over by one of the nurses, who asked me to speak to a family whose daughter had died but they had not been told yet. I had a theoretical idea of how to break bad news to patients, but had not expected to face this scenario on my elective. We found a relatively private area in a corridor and I explained that I was so sorry, but that their ten-year-old daughter had been severely injured in the crash and had died before she had even arrived at the hospital. I winced at my own words. The husband and wife appeared to understand English, but I asked the nurse to check that they had understood. The father thanked me in English, for trying to help and for telling them. He and his wife held each other and walked away in quiet dignity. I was surprised, as I had expected a more dramatic and emotional response to the devastating news. I asked the nurse again if they had understood, as their reaction was subdued. She explained to me that people were not surprised by the loss of a child as it happened so frequently, although not as much as in the past.

The next morning started, for us, in church, before breakfast for once. The singing sounded louder and the prayers seemed more intense than before. The doctors met up after the service and walked to breakfast together. The normal routine and urgent hospital activities needed to carry on as usual, although we had a few more post-operative patients squeezed onto the wards. Two of the most severely injured children were, later that day, transferred by ambulance to the Princess Marina Hospital in Gaborone, where there was a broader range of specialist services and facilities.

Remote Clinics

One of the highlights of my elective was attending to outlying clinics every few weeks in more remote communities. I accompanied Ian in the hospital Toyota minibus to a clinic an hour and a half away, in the Kalahari Desert. We took medicines in a cool box. The dirt roads were heavily rutted and Ian demonstrated his technique for managing the bumps; he would drive at a constant fifty miles per hour so that the wheels bounced up and down into the ruts. It seemed to work but took a bit of courage to reach that speed on such a bumpy path.

The local clinic nurses had brought a few of their more worrying patients into the clinics for us to help. Other patients had travelled a long way already to be seen at these clinics. Some of these had slept for a few nights on the clinic floor. Ian and I split up and worked our way through the waiting patients, with me asking for diagnostic and management help as needed.

Even more nerve-wracking but exciting for me were the two occasions when I was asked to drive to the clinic and see the patients on my own. I was as nervous about the drive as the medical bits, as I had never driven a van before, let alone on a dirt road, at fifty miles an hour. On the first occasion, there was also a sandstorm. These were fairly common along the desert's edge and sometimes lasted a few days. Despite being able to see little but red dust through the windscreen, I managed to find my way, and also managed the waiting patients as best I could.

On my second solo trip out there, I brought a patient back with me. He was in his forties and was jaundiced and unwell. He had been at the clinic for a few days and was unable to stand up. He had no family and there were no proper beds or even full-time staff at the clinic. He lay on the back seat of the minibus on the journey back. I slowed down a bit over the bumps as he was in discomfort, only to find the bumpy ride felt much worse! I sped up and things eased. Ian was a bit bemused that I had brought this chap back, I think, as this was not the norm. The chap, unsurprisingly, had severe liver disease. In his case it was related to chronic liver abscesses and toxin exposure. He was still an inpatient but looked a lot brighter by the time I left to return home. He was often sat in the sun outside the men's ward with some other patients and always nodded at me as I walked past.

One afternoon, I was seeing a patient in the outpatient clinic, when I was interrupted by shouting and screaming coming from the waiting area outside. The clinic aide went out to see what the situation was, then called me from the doorway. 'Come quick,' she said, while waving me over to follow. 'We must go, now!'

I got up and followed her. She shouted to the other aide to get Dr Weil from the other clinic room. The three of us, encouraged by the aide, followed a lady who was by now walking quickly into the warren of huts across the road. We caught up quickly and then followed her into a hut, a few hundred yards from the hospital. It took a few seconds to get used to the darkness in there, but we then saw a young man lying on the floor, adjacent to the open fire in the centre of the room. He was badly burnt and the smell of his burnt clothes and flesh was awful. His eyes were open and he was grunting but not fully conscious. We made sure he was safely clear of the fire and poured cold water from a bowl onto his burns. We had sent the aide back to bring an orderly with a stretcher. We carried him back to the hospital, where we were able to remove his charred clothing and clean him properly. He needed intravenous fluids and painkillers initially, and then several skin graft operations over the next few weeks. It was his mum who had summoned us initially. She'd told us that her son had been having shaking episodes and blackouts for a long time.

The family had sought help from different traditional ('witch' or 'faith') doctors for his condition. This chap was epileptic and was started on anti-convulsant medications during his inpatient stay.

Perhaps surprisingly, severe burns were quite a frequent presentation of epilepsy in Botswana. This is because many people with fits were kept at home as families saw this kind of illness as potentially shameful and also being a sign of some type of curse or inherent badness. Most houses also had large open fires, which were obviously of great potential danger to somebody having a blackout or fit.

Another unusual condition, to me, which I saw while I was there, was of a baby with neonatal tetanus. This condition was still relatively common in Africa in the 1980s. This boy was thought to have contracted the infection from soil, which was frequently applied to the umbilical cord after birth to dry it up. Local healthcare workers tried to discourage mums and traditional midwifes from this practice, but they were often competing with longstanding beliefs and habits. This particular child died. All neonatal deaths are tragic, but this one seemed even more so, as it could have been so easily prevented.

Another problem rarely seen in the UK was snake bites; I saw a girl with particularly severe snake bites on her legs and admitted her. Her bites had become infected, causing her legs to swell massively, and she needed intravenous antibiotics for a few days.

Much of the other emergency work at the hospital related to injuries received in fights, so I spent a lot of time suturing knife and bottle wounds. Botswana was generally not a very violent place, but the younger men often drank home-made booze or spent their spare cash at bottle shops and, as also seen in the UK, high alcohol and testosterone levels often result in late-night drunken scraps.

Time Off

A keen runner, I had completed the Manchester Marathon the week before I came to Botswana (in a time of two hours and fifty-three minutes, for anyone interested). On the nights when I was not on call and had finished before dark, I went for a run. The best route I found was down a dried-up riverbed rather than through the village. Along the edge of the river was extensive fencing and barbed wire because of the border with South Africa. Sometimes the armed guards on the border towers appeared to take a keen interest when I ran past, so I was a bit wary. I also had to hurry, because night fell very quickly so near to the equator.

Afterwards, I would listen to Radio Botswana on my tiny battery-powered radio. The disc jockeys spoke in English and played a limited range of records. They got a copy of *The Nolans' Greatest Hits* while I was there and played one or two tracks from this every night, as well as the more exciting African, guitar-based dance songs. Every night the station closed down at 10.30 p.m. by playing the hymn 'Abide with Me', a song I loved but one that filled me with melancholy as it was played at the FA Cup Final every year. The other channel with reasonable reception was Radio Zimbabwe. At that time, South Africa still operated an apartheid regime. This was obviously an evil and pernicious political system, although the frequent references to it in even the Zimbabwe weather forecasts were amusing.

'The winds will be blowing in from Racist South Africa' and 'Heavy rains from Racist South Africa'.

. . .

I was invited for tea at the doctors' houses a few times and told to pop in again if I needed company. Very kind, although I rarely got much time, especially when on call. The Baxters gave me some lessons in Setswana and also lent me a phrase book. I was also asked to babysit on a few occasions for the Weils; which was a bit challenging when the children woke up, as my O-level German vocabulary did not include the words needed to help me comfort the children, nor overcome their alarm at meeting an anxious English stranger, at night.

Some evenings I wandered into the village after work, often stopping at the local grocery shop for one of their famous 'fat cakes'. These were a savoury deep-fried doughnut ball the size of an apple. I am sure they were very high in calories, which was the point, really, as there was no regular food available in the hospital between lunchtime and the next day's breakfast. I also tried out a local 'bottle shop' on a few occasions. This was a type of bar featuring an off-licence with a group of locals standing outside drinking beer. I met an English teacher, Jake, there on a few occasions: he was volunteering in one of the village schools for a twelve-month period and was glad to catch up on news from the home country.

After I had been there a few weeks, the hospital received a donation of second-hand clothes from a Lutheran charity in the USA: an actual truckload. The hospital superintendent decided that the clothes should be sold off, very cheaply, to villagers, rather than just given away. He decided that this would stop people from just grabbing stuff that they didn't really need or want and the small amount of cash generated could be given to the most needy. Most of the overseas staff and volunteers were roped in to help set up and run this jumble sale on the next Saturday.

We used the hospital classroom and covered all the tables and some borrowed clothes rails with the mountain of donated clothing. It was decided that every item should be sold for the lowest-denomination coin available, with the exception of winter or leather coats, which went for double that fee. The sale was a tremendous success. Every item was sold, including my own jumper after I had rather foolishly left it on the back of a chair. As this was my only jumper, I was a bit hacked off because it was often surprisingly cold at night. I couldn't even buy a replacement item, as I didn't spot it was gone till after the event was over.

I never saw the sweater again, but I did see an awful lot of brightly coloured ski jackets being worn around the village, usually paired with fur-lined trapper hats and the occasional pair of salopettes.

The hospital was set to celebrate its fiftieth anniversary and we were to be visited by the country's health minister. A party and feast were arranged. A whole cow was to be roasted and a variety of stews cooked in cauldron-sized pots over open fires. The cow had been a gift from the village chief, to express his gratitude at the hospital's treatment of his broken leg. All of the inpatients who were well enough sat outside the wards in very smart bright-red dressing gowns. There also appeared to be a lot of local home-brew alcohol around and subsequently a lengthy conga ensued, dancing around much of the hospital grounds late into the night.

On the following weekend, an international fair was taking place on the outskirts of Gaborone in an attempt to persuade the locals to buy overseas products (cars, tractors, machinery). Ian and his wife invited me to go with them. It was a chance to get away from the hospital, enjoy the hospitality and take a look at the local crafts, not to mention the shiny new Land Rovers and tractors.

Somebody behind me shouted out.

'Martin!'

I turned around and saw Sarah, who was another Manchester medic. She and her friends had lived next door to my group at Wythenshawe Hospital during our surgical and medical training in our fourth year. She was with Janet and Dave, who were also UK medical students, and they were all doing their electives at the Princess Marina Hospital in Gaborone. Sarah and Janet were both staying together in a doctor's house in Gaborone. I gave them the mission hospital phone number and they gave me the number for their house phone. After we had arranged to meet up on another weekend, I got my lift back.

On my next free weekend, I got the bus to Gaborone. We went for afternoon tea at the President Hotel in the town centre then did some touristy-type shopping nearby before heading back to their accommodation. This was a large house with a beautiful lawned garden. The family cook brought us drinks. Sarah and Janet seemed a bit bored with their hospital work as they were not allowed to do as much, unsupervised, as I was. They also did not have to do any on-call work. It was all very lovely and luxurious and a bit difficult to tear myself away to catch the bus back to my hospital.

The following weekend they came to see me by bus and on another, we borrowed an old Land Rover and visited some of the historic sites connected with Dr Livingstone, as well as ancient cave paintings. We also began planning a trip into the Okavango Delta.

Okavango

The Okavango is a large inland river delta, which provides a green oasis for plants and wildlife. It's the main tourist attraction in Botswana. The doctors in the mission hospital were very encouraging and practically insisted that all students ought to visit it while in Botswana. This freshwater wetland is world-renowned for its biodiversity, but includes many large mammals such as elephants, hippos and lions. The availability of water in such a relatively confined area, surrounded by deserts, tends to concentrate the animals together and make them easier to see.

Together with four other medical students, two tents and other camping equipment, I flew up to Maun on a twenty-seat plane. From Maun Airport it was then a short flight on a smaller propeller plane into the delta itself, landing on Chief's Island. We had flown over vast herds of elephants and antelopes set in stunning kaleidoscopic scenery. Once at the scrub airstrip, we met up with four local men, who we paid to take us out into the Okavango waterways for five days on three mokoro (canoes made from hollowed-out tree trunks).

The five of us, and all of our camping gear, were spread out across the three boats. We took only dried food with us in order to keep the weight and luggage down: porridge, orange powder, packet soups, rice, teabags and milk powder. The mokoro were poled along in a similar fashion to punts. We set off along the water, between reeds, looking at the spectacular views and amazing birdlife.

A few hours into this idyllic trip, we set up camp in a small wooded glade, just a few yards from the water. The local men showed us how to fish from the boats with nets. They caught a few river bream, which we cooked on an open fire alongside our soup-flavoured rice. The fish tasted nice until we found quite a few live moving worms inside the fish we were eating. We decided to try to overcook any further fish caught on the trip. After tea, and during the sunset, we watched some hippos that were in the water just ten yards offshore. We sat around the fire after that for a while before we settled in our two tents; the two girls in the smaller one and the three lads in the other. The local men slept by the fire.

Our sleep and peace were broken by a tremendous thunderstorm during the night. The jungle was alive with noise from the animals and the thunder, and flashes of lightning. It started raining so heavily that the four local men moved into the girls' tent and turfed the girls out into ours. It was a bit cramped and uncomfortable to say the least, but we eventually awoke to the dawn of another beautiful day. We were taken out early, on foot, to look for animals. We saw lots of antelope and boks and also wildebeest. We were then shown some fresh lion's spoor, meaning footprints. I asked our hosts if they had any weapons in case of close encounters. One of the guys grinned and pulled out a bread knife from his pouch. We were not very reassured by this, to say the least. After a few hours it was getting much hotter and the animals scarcer, so we went back to our camp for breakfast. This was porridge and very-well-done fish.

We packed up and set off again in the boats, deeper into the delta. At one point the hosts punted the mokoro to opposite sides of a lagoon so that we could swim, while they kept their eyes open for hippos and crocodiles. It was lovely and cool, but we didn't hang around too long in there. We saw so much amazing wildlife, but nothing that was too large or threatening or close up.

One interesting encounter was with a honeyguide bird, which kept flying close to us as we floated along. We followed it and then pulled the boats up onto the bank. The bird kept flying back and forth and we all followed it on foot. After about 200 yards into the jungle there was a small clearing and the bird was seen flying near to a beehive, which was hanging from a tree branch. The locals set up a small fire under the nest, while we helped by collecting more twigs and branches. Cue the exit of lots of bees, while we then kept our distance at the other end of the clearing. After ten minutes, the guys went back over and knocked the hive down with some of the larger branches. They broke it open and we all had a share of the honey, including the honeyguide bird, whose portion was left on the sand a few yards away.

We spent the next few days in a similar pattern: early morning foot safari, breakfast, short siesta then moving on to the next camp. We all had a go at poling the mokoro, much to the amusement of our new friends, as we fell overboard or tipped the boats up.

Towards the end of our trip we were running very low on our shared supplies, including the powdered orange. One of the girls had stayed at the camp while we were out walking and was caught helping herself to our last packet when the rest of us arrived back a bit earlier than she expected. She looked suitably embarrassed but then had to cope with the rest of us sulking at her for the last day or so.

We got back to Chief's Island on time and flew out via the small six-seater plane to Maun Airport. Our next flight south was on an old Dakota plane. This was a real treat as it is such an iconic plane; however, there were visible gaps around the doors and it was freezing cold at altitude. We got our sleeping bags down from the overhead shelf and got in these for most of the flight. More fortunately, however, I was allowed to have a look in the cockpit and was amazed at the old-style controls and dials.

The Falls

Three weeks later, Sarah and Janet and I visited the Victoria Falls in Zimbabwe. We went by the night-time steam train to Bulawayo and then hung around there for the day before we got onto the next night train up to The Falls. Bulawayo itself was lovely, with beautiful jacaranda trees in bloom everywhere, particularly in the parks. Also scattered around these parks, and seemingly incongruous and out of place, were numerous defunct tanks and armoured cars that had been left following the recent war.

There was also a large rusted steam train displayed near to a children's playground and I was strangely pleased to read on an attached metal plate that this old train had been made in Patricroft, near my home town, a century earlier. By the park was also an old Portuguese café, which we ate at before walking back to the station. I remember being impressed by the piri-piri chicken meal I had there, wondering why I had never had this lovely dish in the UK. (Nando's appeared to have made a good business decision when they imported their version of Portuguese café style from South Africa in the following decade!)

The trains were marvellous old British-built steam trains and we travelled in lovely compartments with fold-down bunks. Once there, we camped at a proper campsite near to the town centre. On our second day there, we were amazed and amused at a new arrival to the site. This was a large 4x4 truck, which had been fitted out with rows of seats, from which thirty-plus German tourists emerged. The truck was towing a trailer, which carried all of the bunks for the travellers. There were twelve bunks laid side to side down the trailer, with a further two layers added on top, thirty-six in total. All of the bunks had a small window at the far end and access ladders at the nearside. They looked a bit like battery coops or coffins, depending on your mood. The whole set-up was quite claustrophobic and must have been very hot at night. On the plus side, it avoided having to set up a lot of tents at each stop on their trans-African journey.

The Falls were spectacular but, because of the drought in Southern Africa, weren't flowing as they normally did. Highlights of our stay were a sunset safari cruise on the Zambezi river and a safari drive on another evening. We saw some lions on this drive but overall, it was a much less vibrant experience than the Okavango Delta. We also sneaked into the famous Victoria Falls Hotel a few times, with rolled-up towels under our arms, in order to access their pool and grounds. This was a splendid and rather grand hotel. We swam and sunbathed for a few days, all the time serenaded by a fabulous steel drum band playing Glenn Miller songs, mostly 'In the Mood' on heavy repeat. This was the first time I had ever swam or sunbathed overseas, so I thoroughly enjoyed our time there. We also met a few other interlopers by the pool. Some of these were Americans who had just finished their period of voluntary overseas work in the Peace Corps. They had been working in schools in Zimbabwe. We swapped some stories of our time in Africa. The Americans had all had surgery to remove their appendixes before they were allowed to travel abroad on their placements. Not something you would normally have done pre-emptively on the NHS.

Sadly, while we were visiting Victoria Falls, a party of nuns from the mission hospital had visited the Okavango, and one of the nuns was dragged from her tent at night by a lion and was killed. A service was held at the hospital church.

We had, like many others, been oblivious to the real risks of jungle camping until that distressing news.

• • •

It was soon time to return to the UK and I took with me, mostly, fond memories of my time in Botswana and the three months of invaluable medical training: my experiences and responsibilities would have a lasting impact on me. I have never forgotten the doctors, the staff, the friends I found and made, and, most especially, the patients. I arrived there feeling homesick but left having become very fond of the country, and grateful for the opportunity.

There was then, and still is, some debate in the medical community and press about the elective system. Some people feel that the loaning of medical students from rich Western countries to African countries is a remnant of colonial traditions and behaviours. They suggest that it is not fair to allow students to 'practice' and hone their skills on poor, vulnerable foreigners. I engaged in this debate in the letters pages of the *British Medical Journal* (*BMJ*) at that time, on my return home. I personally felt that, overall, medical students offered much-needed help to overworked hospitals, and that they treated patients with appropriate care and respect. Medical students also 'practice' on home patients, but that tends to be called 'training'.

Finals Year

The fifth year was focused on lectures in preparation for our final exams. There was also the small matter of applying for house jobs, the first two six-month pre-registration roles in medicine and surgery. The interviews for these were done on an industrial scale because of the sheer numbers of jobs and applicants to get through. The medical interviews, in particular, were quite an intimidating process. One of mine required sitting in front of twelve medical consultants who took turns asking questions about my CV and career plans. One of the consultants, a keen runner, asked some very specific questions about my running hobby and times, and appeared happy that my claims were real. I was offered a post, dependant on my exam results, of course.

One of my friends, Jagadeep, was interviewed after me and told me that one of the consultants had grilled him about his proclaimed (and genuine) photography hobby. In particular, he asked about a specific new camera. Jagadeep gave it a scathingly poor review, shortly before the consultant revealed that he had just bought one. Jagadeep did not get the post.

My friend, James, applied for a post at a neurosurgical unit and at his interview was asked why he thought that his elective period in Barbados had equipped him for working in that unit. His reply was that lots of Bajans received head injuries from falling coconuts and that he gained valuable experience helping to treat them while on his elective. He did not get the job.

The final exams were tested on the 'whole of medicine' rather than individual subjects or just the final-year subjects. This phrase was used by all lecturers and tutors whenever they were asked what we should focus our revision on. This was a bit daunting but made sense, particularly if you were going to be a patient in the next few years. You would expect your doctors to have a full knowledge of the full medical curriculum rather than just their last year's subjects. Many of the fifth-year lectures were updates and reviews of subjects that we were fairly familiar with, although there were a few extra, newer, subjects.

One of the newer subjects was 'Human Sexual Behaviour'. The final of these lectures was to include video segments featuring demonstrations of these behaviours. The attendance at this final lecture was the highest for nearly five years, with students even having to stand up at the back of the theatre as the benches were full. Many attendees looked a little unfamiliar and we realised that quite a few of them were hospital staff members, mostly porters, who had sneaked in. This was pre-internet. The videos featured enthusiastic Californian actors demonstrating vigorous straight and gay sex. Most of the audience had not seen anything like that before, at least on-screen. There were quite a lot of complaints and questions afterwards, particularly from the more religiously minded students, wondering why we had to be exposed to 'pornography'. Most of the other students had been amused or entertained. Some of the hospital porters tried to find out the date for the next year's film show.

Our finals included viva sessions in which we were questioned by specialists about real patients on the wards, or those with rarer conditions and clinical signs who had come in especially for the exams. One of the patients I examined appeared to have frostbite, which was unusual even for the North during June. He had underlying vascular disease, but I correctly guessed that he must also be homeless to have been sufficiently exposed to develop frostbite. Another patient had developed an apparent occupational repetitive strain injury of the left forearm. I was asked to conjecture what occupation this young woman may be in. I spotted that her nails were much longer on her right hand than on her left, so thought she may have been a musician, specifically a guitarist. It turned out that she was a violinist, so I guess that I was close enough, as I later found out that I had passed that particular exam.

We found out our results one stressful morning in the medical school, when we were all handed our envelopes. I passed, as did all my immediate friends and tutorial group members. Medical degrees tend to be awarded as professional degrees in the UK, so are a pass or fail, rather than First or a 2:1, for example. Most seemed a bit excited to tell their families and there were very long queues at the payphones in the lobby for students ringing home and saying, 'You can call me Doctor.'

My next stop after that was at the bank to request a loan so I could buy a car: essential for getting to my forthcoming hospital posts, but also because I just wanted a car and could finally get one. It was a second-hand brown three-door Ford Escort, which I loved, despite its plain looks. Its first proper use was on a trip to the Lakes a few days after purchase, for a hiking and youth hostel trip.

I was due to start work as a pre-registration house officer on the first of August, but was rung by the consultant asking if I could start as a locum two weeks early, so that my predecessor could go on leave. It was assumed that I would not say no, so I didn't.

House Officer Year

I had no idea quite how much house officers did. I was attached to a respiratory team, which was part of the general medical and geriatrics rota for out of hours. The weekdays were occupied by doing any job required for the respiratory patients of Dr Hulley. This included arranging all investigations, putting in catheters, inserting chest drains, writing prescriptions, putting up drips, taking blood and performing all required intravenous injections.

Day one. I was bleeped by a nurse at 5 p.m.

'The INRs are back.'

I had no idea what this meant, but went to the ward. It turned out that INR* blood test results came back to each ward in late afternoon and required a doctor to look at it, in order to adjust the patients' warfarin dose. I didn't know how to adjust the dose, so rang my SHO.† He had finished so I then rang an on-call SHO for advice. He was kind enough to help by giving me a few simple tips. Before I put the phone down, I had received messages to ring another four wards to go and do their warfarin dosing, too. I finished that task at 6.30 p.m. and looked forward to going home. My bleep rang again: apparently, there were three patients being admitted to that ward following domiciliary visits by Dr Hulley. I clerked them in as best I could, without knowing what his plans or expectations were for them. None were acutely

---

* International normalised ratio. A measure of coagulation levels used in order to adjust the dose of anticoagulant (usually warfarin). Patients were given a certain range for their INR to be in, which varied, dependent on their diagnosis.

† Senior house officer.

ill, but I suspected he had admitted them for further investigation. I finished at 8.30 p.m.

The next day was a duty day. That meant that I would work the ordinary working day from 8 a.m. and then be on call all of that night, followed by working the normal next day until 5 p.m., or perhaps 8.30 p.m. if the consultant admitted a few extras. On call, in such a busy hospital, meant working pretty much full-on for the whole of the duty time and certainly no time to sleep. Duty days there were divided into admissions or ward cover.

Admissions meant dealing with the GP medical and geriatric referrals, as well as the same groups of patients either admitted from A&E or seen in that department. There could be as many as twenty admissions overnight, or thirty if it was a weekend day. My colleague, Nigel, was my SHO and dealt with the GP admission request phone calls. He had a few years of medical experience and had the authority, which I did not have, to discharge patients, including those we were invited to see in A&E. He found acute medicine a bit stressful and was planning a career in radiology, hoping to avoid having to talk to patients as much.

He told me that he had a recurring dream on the nights before duty sessions, of standing on the fortified walls of the hospital, trying to repel the hordes of patients with hot oil, while the patients were trying to beat their way in with battering rams.

Many of the patients were very ill and required a lot of input to diagnose, treat and monitor. Other interventions included fitting pacemakers to patients with heart block.*

There were eleven medical wards as well as the coronary care unit (CCU) and intensive care units (ICUs), and ward cover meant covering these wards overnight and at weekends. There

---

* When the electrical impulses that control the beating of the heart muscle are disrupted. This is potentially life-threatening, particularly when it has just happened after a myocardial infarction or heart attack.

were always other more experienced doctors also working on the last two units, but many of the mundane jobs were still passed on to the house officer. The other wards required the houseman to put all drips in, and to give all the intravenous (IV) drugs, and take all bloods at nights and weekends.

Nowadays, nurses are trained and expected to do many of these jobs. The IV drugs in particular were quite an onerous task: often needing visits to all eleven wards at midnight and at 6 a.m. just to make up and administer the required antibiotics alone. Sometimes the ward nurses would ring at 4 a.m. to remind you not to forget to come at 6 a.m. and 'so you don't fall asleep'. Fat chance of that.

My first weekend on call lasted from Saturday at 9 a.m. until Monday at 8 p.m. I got no sleep at all in that time, and was really struggling with fatigue and concentration by the Sunday evening. I remember getting visual hallucinations of spiders running around at the edges of my vision while examining a patient on a geriatric ward at 2 a.m. on the Monday; not to be confused with seeing hundreds of actual live cockroaches in the underpass on the way to the ward, of course.

The working hours were ridiculous and dangerous and were thankfully changed a few years later to bring them into line with European working time directives. I was on a one-in-three rota in that post, which meant working the standard forty-hour week as well as a third of the other available hours, so therefore eighty-two hours a week. Other posts I did later on were on a one-in-two basis, meaning 104 average hours a week, but being as many as 144 hours on the weeks in which a weekend duty was included. I was seldom able to get any sleep at all on my shifts due to the busyness of the particular hospital departments I worked in. I understand that when these type of shifts were first agreed and undertaken that doctors often did get the time to sleep: the change in this relating to increased activity and newer treatments, which were available and expected.

An example would be the treatment of myocardial infarctions or heart attacks. In the fifties and sixties, treatment for these conditions was limited to administering morphine and putting patients to bed, hoping they survived. As more treatments, such as IV drug infusions and pacemakers, became available, these patients would be monitored and treated throughout the night. The rotas persisted well beyond their safe status, in part due to the fact that doctors were only paid a third of their normal hourly rate for these overtime hours, even at night or bank holidays. No hospital authority was going to volunteer to pay extra doctors at full pay when they could compel their current staff to work for a third of their usual pay. Junior doctors were paid less than any other hospital employees during weekends or bank holidays.

Thankfully, the changed working time directives brought down the allowable working hours for medical staff, although they are often still encouraged to agree to work outside these limits. The downside of reducing hours is that junior doctors are now exposed to less, unsupervised, out-of-hours time, so often have less experience and confidence in managing acute medical conditions. The lot of a junior doctor remains very stressful, though, because hospitals feel overloaded and overwhelmed pretty much all of the time and, as patients, we are all less accepting of unsatisfactory and delayed care than previous generations may have been. All of this, in addition to the large erosion of comparative pay levels, means perhaps it's little wonder that this has recently led to sustained periods of strikes by these doctors.

Because we were working across so many different wards, it was difficult to form any particular attachments to any one of the wards or nursing teams, but it remained a good idea to listen to the nurses, who had far more experience in dealing with patients in their specialities than junior doctors did, as well as a better understanding of the needs of the specific patient you were reviewing together. They would also help to explain procedures that they had seen but you hadn't. As I have already mentioned, it was never a stupid thing to ask the nurse or sister what they felt you should do with a given patient and seldom a bad thing to actually do what they expected, unless you had a strong opinion to the contrary.

Plus, you got more cups of coffee and biscuits offered to you when you were known to be approachable, rather than arrogant and aloof.

Big Bang

My consultant, Dr Hulley, was a respiratory physician. On duty days, we would admit all medical emergencies under his care, but otherwise he would only admit patients with chest problems onto the 'chest' wards. These wards were old-fashioned Nightingale wards, although there were a few one-bed side wards at the top of both the male and female wards. These were usually occupied by patients with lung diseases, most often different types of chronic obstructive pulmonary disease (COPD), although these were still broadly known as 'bronchitis' or 'emphysema' in those days.

Mr Towell was such a patient and was staying in one of the single rooms in the male ward. He was suffering from an infective exacerbation of his COPD and was receiving intravenous antibiotics, nebulised medications, oral antibiotics, oral steroids, as well as oxygen therapy via a mask. He was a smoker, like ninety-nine per cent of such patients, but was currently bed-bound, so was unable to access the day room for a smoke, which was still allowed in the 1980s. I was on the main ward taking arterial blood samples from another COPD patient, when there was a very loud bang from nearby. Several nurses and I ran up the ward to see what had happened. The main corridor was clear, so we looked into the side room. There was a strong burning smell but no obvious fire.

Mr Towell was sat up in bed with a blackened face and burnt eyebrows.

'Sorry, love,' said Mr Towell to the nearest nurse. 'I couldn't wait. I was dyin' for a fag.'

He had lit up a cigarette and popped it through one of the holes in his face mask. Pure oxygen and fire tend to like each other very much and had exploded. Luckily, Mr Towell was not badly injured and, even more luckily, the small explosion had not spread to the piped oxygen in his room or the rest of the hospital.

He may well have been dying for a fag but, on that particular day, he came perilously close to dying from it, too.

Learning to Live

I was working at my medical house officer post. A lady of ninety-two was admitted on a Saturday afternoon, from A&E, because of her abdominal pain. Patients with problems like this would ordinarily be looked after by surgeons and be admitted to a surgical ward, but the surgeons had reviewed her and decided that she had no need of surgery. They had not come up with a definitive diagnosis, but as she was frail and elderly and not well enough to be discharged, she was transferred onto an acute medical ward.

I was called to clerk her in, which meant: taking a medical history; performing an appropriate examination; coming up with a putative diagnosis; arranging initial investigations and treatment plans – the latter after speaking to a more senior doctor if you were the lowest-ranked house officer in the firm.

This lady, Joan, was groaning in pain and found it difficult to speak, but I had some surprising help from her sister.

Her identical twin sister, Margaret.

Margaret was fit and well and remarkably chipper and cheerful, especially given her age. She was able to answer pretty much all of the questions I had and I was near to completing the history-taking, when she told me, as an aside: 'You know, of course, that she's got cancer?'

'Sorry, no, what kind of cancer?' I asked, not having read any reference at all to this in her A&E and surgical notes.

'We don't know. The doctor didn't say,' she replied, fairly nonchalantly.

I was even more baffled and asked, 'When was this?'

'Ooh, when she was about forty. Our GP told me to look after her, so I have done.'

My curiosity and incredulity were awoken further, and I asked, 'And then what happened?'

'We just put her to bed and looked after her. Still do.'

I had to ask: 'Did you not think he might have been wrong with the diagnosis, given that she has already lived another fifty-odd years since?'

'Oh no, I'm sure he was right, doctor. She just learnt to live with it.'

That is certainly one way of coping with cancer, I suppose. It is hard to imagine such touching, and inappropriate, levels of faith in doctors nowadays, which is perhaps as well.

Joan was diagnosed with, and treated for, diverticulitis, which is an unpleasant bowel infection or inflammation.

Margaret visited her every day and sat with her for the duration of allowed visiting hours until her discharge five days later. She shook her head a little every time she caught sight of me, still having not forgiven me for my implied criticism of her old doctor, and casting doubt on her fixed belief and half a lifetime of caring so lovingly for her sister.

Remember Me?

During a ward round with Dr Hulley, I noticed a vicar sat by a patient's bed, further down on the left. As our entourage approached, he kept looking up anxiously towards us. Finally, as we stopped by the patient in the next bed, he stood up and walked over towards the notes trolley. He extended his hand towards the consultant and spoke loudly.

'Dr Hulley! Remember me?'

He obviously didn't, and peered over his half-moon reading glasses towards the vicar. He was also, obviously, a little irritated at being interrupted, but polite enough to look interested and try.

'Oh, yes, of course, it's err …'

The vicar quickly put him out of his misery. 'Reverend West. You looked after my wife last year. She asked me to thank you if I saw you.'

Dr Hulley smiled and spoke again. 'Oh yes, I remember. Rose. Rose West.'

Reverend West looked mortified, as did the rest of us, stood by the trolley, and he said, 'No, that's the murderer!'

Dr Hulley answered swiftly, 'No. Murderess.' As if correcting the sex of the killer made his confusion less shocking.

He then walked off quickly, leaving the open-mouthed vicar aghast in the middle of the ward. We all scurried off hurriedly and followed Dr Hulley to the next patient. I sneaked a look back at the vicar, who had remained where we left him. The nursing sister saw me looking and we shared a mutual grimace. I wonder if Reverend West ever told his wife that he had bumped into Dr Hulley and passed on her thanks – or the doctor's reply …

Surgical Posting

My six-month surgical house-officer post was in Oldham. The posting was with a general surgical unit. Most of their work related to abdominal surgery, but also out-of-hours responsibility for other surgical problems. One late-night operation was an appendicectomy on a ninety-year-old: an unusual procedure at that age. The expectation on going to theatre was that this gentleman's abdominal pain and sepsis was caused by a colonic cancer but, unexpectedly, the cause turned out to be an inflamed and perforated appendix. Unfortunately, the patient received damage to their spleen during the surgery by the registrar, Mr Edwards, and required a splenectomy. At the ward round the following morning, our consultant, Mr Hurst, was surprised at this unfortunate surgical incident, as the patient's spleen was some distance from the appendix, and asked the registrar, 'How did you manage to nick the spleen?'

Mr Edwards replied, with a straight face, 'It was very difficult, sir.'

Mr Hurst looked confused at the sarcastic reply, then appeared deep in thought for a few moments, shook his head and walked to the next patient on the round.

My most difficult task was usually just staying awake. I felt envious of the patients lying in bed, surrounded by grapes and daytime TV, while recovering from routine operations.

I wished I could swap places with them.

I didn't wish to be ill or have any serious health problems.

I just wanted a rest and some sleep.

'She Knows Her Onions'

Next up for me, but still in Oldham, was a senior house officer post in the Geriatric department. I would spend six months in this role but would continue working in the same hospital for the next two years as part of my GP training. The lead consultant, Dr Mehti, had started this department, and had gained respect for his holistic and practical care of older people. The speciality was relatively new and unestablished, and many consultants in the field were physicians who were more used to working with younger people and then transferred that type of care to older patients. This was not always necessarily appropriate.

Several patients in their nineties were treated with aggressive protocols for managing heart failure, whereas they and their families may have been better served by some consideration to their age, frailty and dignity. In contrast, on one particular ward round with Dr Mehti, we reviewed the care of a chap in his late seventies. He had had a relatively mild stroke and was nearly ready for discharge, following medical treatment and rehabilitation on the ward. His wife was sitting by the bed. Dr Mehti suggested that the gentleman could be discharged soon, as he was mobile and, mostly, self-caring. The wife shook her head a little and said she wasn't happy that he'd had a stroke.

Dr Mehti spoke again. 'Madam, you married your husband for better or worse. This is worse. You should now allow your husband back to his home, with you.'

The wife responded to this approach, with, 'Yes, Dr Mehti.'

The ward sister and I made notes of all the jobs we needed to do in order to complete the discharge, while Dr Mehti scribbled some comments in the patient's notes, leaning on the ward trolley. He asked the sister which district nurse would be visiting this gentleman when he arrived home. She told him it was Dawn, who used to work on this ward. This information led Dr Mehti to speak to the wife again. 'Madam, your district nurse is excellent. I trained her myself. She knows her onions …' He paused and then added, 'Backwards.'

The wife looked more reassured still and thanked Dr Mehti. The sister gave her a hug before re-joining us as we moved on to the next bed.

At this time there were still many 'geriatric' patients with severe chronic disease staying in long-term beds, many of them also suffering from severe end-stage dementia. Nowadays, these patients would be cared for in elderly persons homes (EPHs) in the community or even in nursing homes. I was fast-bleeped to a collapse on one of these wards and I arrived there at the same time as an anaesthetist, who had also been summoned urgently. A lady was choking on a boiled sweet. We managed to retrieve this sweet and restore her breathing. She was sat back up in bed, unable to communicate verbally with us, having had a severe stroke many years ago, but was able to smile at us and the nurses. I thanked the anaesthetist and said I would write up the details in the patient's notes. The notes were open on the desk at the nurse station. I wrote up the details of our intervention, then looked back over the page at the last medical entry in her records. This was from three years before and read, 'Choked on boiled sweet. Sweet retrieved. Not to have boiled sweets again.' I closed the notes and noticed that there was also a warning on the front to avoid boiled sweets.

I asked a nurse if this lady had many visitors and was told that she had never had any. Presumably, the sweets were ones donated to the ward by other patients' visitors.

I walked back to the acute wards, feeling sorry for this poor old lady whose only visitors appeared to be doctors summoned to her choking episodes, three years apart.

Male Nurse

Paul was a male nurse working on one of the geriatric wards. He liked to entertain staff and patients with colourful stories from his past. He wore rubber gloves, which was unusual.

I asked him why and he said, 'I don't want to catch anything. Who'd believe I'd caught AIDs from work if I ever got it?'

Being gay in Salford during the 1960s, when he was first active, had also been risky. Homosexuality was still illegal in the UK until 1967 and was still marginalised well beyond that time. Paul had been arrested a number of times while meeting up with other men in public toilets for sex. On one occasion, he was offered sexuality conversion therapy as an alternative to a prison sentence after being found guilty of public indecency.

The therapy consisted of attending a course run with monitoring by a psychiatrist. Paul and the others on his course were shown a series of photographs, projected onto a screen. These were of attractive, naked young men. So far, so good, you might think; however, Paul and the others had devices strapped to their penises. These devices detected any increases in the width of their penises due to the development of erections and then administered an electric shock to the same area, as a type of aversion therapy.

I asked Paul if this effected any changes in his sexuality and he suggested that it might have made him more 'kinky', as he started getting off on the shocks as well as the pictures.

A&E

My next posting was as an SHO in the A&E department. One of the great things about this was being part of a proper team all working in one unit. Most of my time as a junior doctor until then had been spent working across different wards, sometimes as many as ten during a single shift. Work was also usually completed alone, apart from the patients, of course, and you were rarely sat down long enough to get to know any ward staff, or even the other doctors on your team, or 'firm', as they were known. Working as an SHO in A&E was very different, with shifts often matching the nursing ones, so we were therefore able to build up a proper team relationship with them, for once. The lead consultant was keen on training and most of us attended the regular Thursday lunchtime lectures that he arranged. Staff who were working on night shifts were still encouraged to attend and the on-duty staff were also able to attend, as GP locums were paid to cover the department for the duration of the sessions.

The teamwork extended outside work, too. We shared nights out and all even attended the wedding of the senior sister. At another time we had taken part in a local sponsored fancy-dress walk. This walk also included drinking a little too much beer than was healthy or sensible. So much so that I was still embarrassingly hungover on the following Sunday morning, when I was the only doctor on duty for a three-hour period. During this time I felt increasingly nauseous and needed to run to the loo to be sick in between seeing each patient. At 11 a.m., my colleague, Stuart, came on duty. He took one look at me and said I looked dreadful. He suggested that he put up a glucose drip to rehydrate and energise me a little. I agreed, glad to have a lie down for half an hour, too. I felt much better after the infusion and was able to work normally till my shift finished at teatime. It was a very effective hangover cure but I was, thankfully, never in a position to require nor request this dramatic treatment again.

Shooting

We had been given advance notice by the ambulance service that a patient was on his way to our A&E, having been shot in the neck. The police were also on their way, hoping to interview him after his treatment. He was a seventy-eight-year-old gentleman and, on arrival, the crew were holding some bloodstained swabs against the right side of his neck, just below the ear. There was not much active bleeding and he was haemodynamically stable with no signs of physical shock. This meant that his blood pressure and pulse were within a normal range and it looked like he had not lost very much blood. I removed the dressing and there was a small circular wound beneath his ear, with only gentle rather than heavy bleeding when the pressure was taken off.

The police had arrived by this point and told us that they thought this man had been shot by an air rifle, as several witnesses had reported seeing teenagers in the area with such a weapon. They had been seen shooting at birds in the park. They had not been found at that time. The nature of the wound and condition of the patient certainly supported a pellet rather than a bullet wound. The poor chap was really upset, though, and had been crying.

He said, 'I managed to get through the war without the Germans hitting me and some toerags shoot me while I'm going for a walk!'

I assured him he was going to be OK and that we would sort him out. He told me that he was not in pain, just angry. We all felt sympathy and anger on his behalf. The police had contacted his family and they were now on their way. I spoke to the duty surgical registrar and asked if he would come and have a look at the wound, but he was already tied up in theatre. He suggested I just anaesthetise the area and clean it properly, before extracting the pellet if I could. I did what he asked and found the pellet fairly easily; it was not very deep, so I retrieved it with forceps and handed it to the police in a pot. Fortunately, there was no major structural damage, despite the presence of important arteries and nerves in the vicinity of the pellet.

I finished cleaning the small wound and sutured it. His two children arrived shortly after and took him home after he had been given a cup of tea and been fussed over appropriately by the nurses in the department.

The local newspaper had a short article about this incident the following day. I was most impressed at the dramatic headline:

DOCTORS FIGHT TO SAVE THE LIFE OF WAR VETERAN AFTER SHOOTING

I cut out the article and pinned it up on the A&E common-room noticeboard. Nobody else was impressed. Several nurses tutted and then ignored it. My fifteen minutes of fame had passed, unnoticed.

One Friday teatime, I was sat at the main nursing desk, writing in patients' notes and talking to Julie, one of the nursing sisters, when a couple of people approached the desk. It was the hospital matron with a senior manager in tow. The matron introduced the manager to Julie and explained that they were struggling to manage nurse numbers in the hospital for the evening and later night shifts. They were keen to borrow some of the A&E nurses to help on the wards.

Julie was a little reluctant. 'No,' she said.

'Well, what if it stays quiet tonight?' tried the manager, being both brave and foolish at the same time.

'What do you mean?' Julie asked.

'Well, how many patients will be coming in tonight?' he asked.

'What?' asked Julie.

'How many patients will come in tonight?' he said patiently, pen poised over his A4 clipboard.

'It's a casualty department. How do I know?' said Julie.

'I know that, but you must have an idea. What's the average?' he pressed on.

'About eighty patients between six and midnight, I think,' she said through gritted teeth.

'Right. Now we're getting somewhere. How many patients do you expect tonight?' He raised his pen again.

'OK. Anything between none and two hundred. It depends on whether we get a plane crashing into a coachload of pensioners or not. It's a fucking casualty department!' Very much louder now.

'There's no need for that,' said the matron. 'We're only trying to help.'

'Well, you can help me by buggering off and mithering somebody else. We need all of our nurses and we need them straightaway when they're needed. None of their nurses come down here when we ask for help. They're too busy eating chocolates.' With that, Julie turned her back on them and walked back to the desk. A few minutes later, she whispered to me, without looking up, 'Have they gone yet?'

They had.

Blackout

A patient was brought in, by an ambulance crew, on a stretcher. He was a man in his mid-thirties and was semi-conscious. Fortunately, a work colleague was with him to tell us what had happened. He had already given the story to the 999 call handler and then the ambulance crew and was fairly well-practised by the time he was talking to me.

'He's epileptic and he's had a fit at work.'

'Did he hurt himself as far as you could tell?' I asked.

'No, he just slumped down and shook a bit, but he didn't injure himself.'

Another question: 'Is he on any medications, do you know?'

'Yes, but they're in his locker at work,' he replied. 'This has happened a few times and he usually comes round a bit quicker than this,' he added, helpfully, and then, 'He doesn't work with any machinery 'cos of this.'

I thanked him and he was then ushered to the reception window to give some more personal information about his colleague.

I examined the patient. His observations were all normal except for his reduced state of consciousness; not that unusual for some people to suffer from a temporary postictal drowsiness after an epileptic fit. He was placed in a safe recovery position and a nurse stayed with him in a cubicle. We expected him to come round gradually. The nurse was checking his observations regularly and I popped in to check on him every ten minutes or so, as did the charge nurse and one of the A&E consultants. We all became a bit more concerned as time went on, as he was not coming round and had become a bit more sweaty. It was time to

start some investigations, such as blood tests and also an ECG.*
The first and quickest blood test was a finger-prick blood-glucose
level. This gave a very low reading, so we initiated a dextrose (a
type of sugar) infusion. The patient then came round and sat up
pretty quickly, thankfully. He was able to speak freely after a
few minutes.

'Are you diabetic?' I asked him.

'Yes,' he replied.

'Do you also have epilepsy?'

'No. Diabetes is bad enough, thanks.'

I established that he was a Type 1 diabetic and that he'd been
struggling recently to try to get the right dosage and timing for
his insulin injections. He'd had quite a few 'hypos' (hypogly-
caemic/low blood sugar episodes) recently. Some of these had
happened at work and he did not always have enough warning
or self-awareness to deal with them in time. The laboratory tests
confirmed that his blood sugar had been very low, but that all
other bloods were fine, as was his ECG. The charge nurse spoke
to this chap's specialist diabetic nurse, who was based in the
hospital. She popped down to talk to him and discuss amending his treatment. I suggested that he should consider getting
an SOS bracelet, so that he may get faster treatment if he were
acutely unwell again in the future.

While this conversation was going on, I spied his work
colleague, who was sat at the front of the waiting room. I gestured
for him to pop back into the department, into a more private area.

'Did you say your mate was epileptic?' I asked.

'Yes,' he replied.

'Are you sure you didn't mean diabetic?'

---

* Electrocardiogram. This is a relatively simple test that is used to
check up on the heart's rhythm and electrical activity. The sensors for
this are attached to the skin of the chest and limbs.

'That's it! Diabetic. That's the one,' he said confidently and then, 'I knew it was something like that.'

I explained to him that the two conditions were nothing like each other but left it at that. His misinformation had delayed his friend's diagnosis and treatment. Had his friend been found collapsed somewhere and without any other information, we would have done his blood tests immediately on his arrival at the unit. A period of prolonged hypoglycaemia can be extremely dangerous. This chap seemed to have escaped unscathed, however, with no great thanks to his colleague.

Child

One of the best things about working in A&E was the variety of work, with complete unpredictability of the next patient's illness or problem. You had no idea what you would see or treat next. An exception to this was when an ambulance was en route to the unit and was carrying a seriously ill or injured patient. Usually we would then receive a call from the central control or the crew themselves, warning us and offering an estimated arrival time. If there were multiple casualties, say from a significant road traffic accident (RTA), the hope was that we could also alert a few other relevant speciality teams to try to get them to A&E before the patient(s) arrived, as well as the other A&E doctors and nurses working elsewhere in the department.

On one such occasion, we received warning of the imminent arrival of an eleven-year-old lad who had collapsed while playing football. The crew had been in attendance with him for a while before they alerted us that they were on the way and expected to be with us in eight minutes. Another junior doctor and two nurses were waiting with me as the ambulance arrived. The crew ran into the department, pushing the unfortunate lad on the gurney.* The crew looked distressed and the older of the two was shaking his head.

He said, 'He's still got a weak pulse, but he's made no respiratory effort for over an hour now.'

I asked the nurse to put out a crash call,† and I also shouted to another nurse who was attending to another nearby patient,

---

* A wheeled stretcher.

† An emergency request for the crash team to attend and try to resuscitate a collapsed patient; often following a cardiac arrest.

'Please get the sister and a consultant. We need an anaesthetist too – quickly!'

I was usually able to avoid panicking while at work, or at least hide it from others. My technique was to count to three and take a deep breath in and out, while trying to look outwardly relaxed. Not this time. There was no time to even try. I needed to intubate* this child so we could get some oxygen into his circulation. Intubation was a great skill and it would have been a great benefit to have had lots of practice at this technique, which I didn't have. Specifically, I had never intubated a child before. I needed to try, as nobody else had turned up yet. We got the lad into the right position and the nurse passed me the correct size plastic tube while I turned the laryngoscope† on and hooked the curved end into the boy's throat. My panic subsided – I managed to see the vocal cords and was able to pass the tube through. We were in business. The tube was connected to the oxygen supply and we were able to bag‡ the lad and get some oxygen flowing into his lungs and on out through his arteries. We were then able to set up drips and connect our ECG leads and try to assess the situation better. By this stage, other more senior doctors started to arrive and take over. The lad was stabilised, but the big unspoken worry was how much brain damage must have been done while he was not breathing spontaneously for such a long period.

The ambulance crew had done an amazing job to sustain him. One of them had to drive while the other kept the boy alive

---

* Passing a tube into a patient's trachea to allow control of the unconscious patient's ventilation/breathing.

† An instrument used to examine the patient's larynx and to help guide a tube into their trachea in order to assist their breathing. It is an L-shaped device with a handle, a light and a curved metal blade.

‡ To 'bag' is to manually squeeze a small rubber bag to push air or oxygen through a tube and into the patient's lungs.

in the back. At this time, none of our local ambulance crews were trained as paramedics. Nowadays, you would expect paramedics to attend a similar incident and perhaps they may expect to call on an air ambulance as backup to assist them: this service was also unavailable in those days.

The A&E consultant arrived and made his own assessment and then awaited the arrival of the boy's parents. He asked me to contact the on-call anaesthetist (who had still not arrived yet) in order to request a transfer of the lad to the Intensive Care Unit (ICU). I bleeped him. A rather angry anaesthetic registrar, Dr Wolff, rang back. I explained the situation and asked for him to accept the lad for transfer onto ICU.

He became even angrier and said, 'We are incredibly busy up here and don't want some brain-dead kid blocking up a bed for a week before we can turn the machines off!'

Crikey. Talk about unexpected and insensitive. I didn't normally argue with more senior doctors, but I felt emboldened and had, I thought, the moral high ground on this occasion.

I said, 'Well, you can tell his parents that when they get here, as they don't even know yet. Shall we keep him here for a week instead?'

'Don't they know what's happened?' he asked.

I sensed a little backtracking and replied, 'No, I don't think so. All they know is he collapsed playing football. They dropped him off, fit and well, at school this morning.' I made the last bit up, but it was likely to have been true.

He said, 'Err, OK. I'll come down and have a look at him.'

Dr Wolff saw him and, somewhat reluctantly, allowed his transfer upstairs to ICU. He was, of course, sadly correct about the poor lad staying on ICU for a week or so. I popped up every day to see to see how he was doing. Tragically, and also as predicted, the boy never regained consciousness. After an appropriate delay for proper testing and retesting of his brain function, his parents agreed to the removal of his life-support systems and said their goodbyes. An awful tragedy.

A few years later, I met up with Dr Wolff again. He had switched from his intended career in anaesthetics and onto the same GP training scheme that I was on. One lunchtime I reminded him that we had spoken and met before, when dealing with the poor lad mentioned previously, and that he had initially been obnoxious on the phone. He said he did not remember the call but admitted that he had struggled in that posting. A few years later, I heard that he had sadly passed away in his thirties, due to the physical complications of long-term alcohol abuse.

SHO Post 3 – Paediatrics

My next role was in a six-month posting as a paediatrics SHO, which also included some work on the child psychiatry unit. The whole posting was naturally very different to adult medicine but equally as challenging. There was also the obvious matter of dealing with that most precious of materials: children. From a personal perspective, things appeared a bit worse, as I was now working on a one-in-two rota, but at least there were chances to get some sleep on many of the duty nights.

On the general paediatrics wards, my roles were similar to my previous posts, which included clerking and admitting the patients. Here, there was generally good support from more experienced SHOs and a registrar, although they were often both away from the ward at the same time, dealing with newborns in the delivery suites or the special care baby unit (SCBU).

Early on in this posting, I clerked an eighteen-month-old boy who had been admitted by his GP because of suspected meningitis. The boy required an urgent lumbar puncture before I could administer intravenous penicillin. It was important to do it in that order wherever possible, as giving an antibiotic before taking the sample could potentially make the sample unhelpful. As I had never seen a lumbar puncture on a child, I bleeped my seniors to help, thinking they were both at the nearby SCBU. One was, and was dealing with a very ill newborn baby, but the other was at the other local hospital, helping with a child who had been injured in an RTA. The usual learning and teaching method for new procedures in medicine was an informal rule of three: that is, see one, do one, teach one. On this occasion, I had to skip step one and just get on with it. The procedure went well, despite my nervousness, and I was able to give the penicillin quickly thereafter. The lab tests on the sample later confirmed the diagnosis. The boy recovered well, as did his older sister, who was also admitted with meningitis on the following day.

We had two long-stay children on the ward when I started, both effectively kept alive by life support machines and also IV fluids. They were both still there when I finished. Both had been born with metabolic diseases, inherited from their parents who were cousins, as was often custom and tradition in their communities. I understand that this tradition persists in these communities, and the tragedy of such severe illnesses is still having an impact on the families and also on the health services covering the communities. The preventable nature of the diseases adds to the level of the tragedy.

My work on the child psychiatry unit was mostly in providing medical rather than any direct psychiatric care. There were two child psychiatrists attached to the unit and several psychother-apists, as well as child psychiatric nurses and play therapists. There were only a few children actually staying on the ward long term. Most of the children who presented at the outpatients or for short-term assessments had no formal psychiatric conditions but had behavioural problems associated with chaotic or non-existent parenting. Many of their parents were addicts or had severe psychiatric diseases of their own.

Of some interest on the unit were case conferences that I was invited to attend, mostly as an observer rather than active contrib-utor. The pace and intensity of work on the ward and at these meetings was a world away from the usual paediatric wards. Very little seemed to get achieved: in fact, half of the meeting time was spent by social workers trying to find matching windows in their diaries for the next meeting. One case that came up at every meeting was that of the longest-stay patient on the unit, Craig.

He was a nine-year-old lad. His mum was a heroin addict with Scottish heritage. His biological dad was from Cyprus but had not had much involvement in the lad's life so far. His long-term stepfather was from Lebanon. Social services were keen to place Craig with a foster or adoptive family, and were equally keen that all elements of his heritage and upbringing should be represented in his new family. That is, Scottish, Cypriot and Lebanese. It was no wonder that he had been stuck on the ward for so long, despite there being a few families who were actually interested in adopting him, without possessing the essential household ethnic mix, of course. I hope he's not still on the ward.

Study Leave

While I was on the paediatrics rotation, I often had to provide cover for some of the career paediatric doctors. They, not unreasonably, often took study leave to attend courses relevant to their training. I decided to try to organise some study leave of my own and spoke to a local GP, Dr Astley.

I had met Dr Astley while I was working in A&E. He sometimes locumed in the department while all the A&E staff had training lectures from the consultant. I asked if I could sit in with him at his surgery for a few weeks. He said that I could, but I should be aware that it was not a training practice and that he was 'different' to other GPs.

I arranged the placement, much to everyone's bafflement and amusement, as none of the previous GP-training SHOs had taken such study leave. I really enjoyed sitting in on surgeries and home visiting, getting a proper sense of the pace and working style of General Practice. Dr Astley had a very broad Lancashire accent and was quite blunt with his patients. He was not immensely dissimilar to Les Dawson, a brilliant Northern comedian of the time, particularly famed for his deadpan delivery. The patients loved him.

I was sitting in with him when a rather small and timid middle-aged lady came in for her consultation.

'Hello, Edith,' he said as she neared the chair.

'Hello, Dr Astley,' she replied, sitting down.

Dr Astley continued, 'I was driving down Manchester Road last week, and I saw somebody with such a miserable face that I felt like mounting the pavement and running her over. Do you know who that was?'

She shook her head and replied softly, 'No.'

'You!' he said more loudly.

'Ooh, Dr Astley, you are funny,' she said while giggling. The rest of the consultation started and finished without either of them referring to his introductory remarks.

She left, appearing satisfied with the outcome.

As the door closed, Dr Astley turned to me and said, 'I meant it, but nobody seems to take me seriously.' I muttered that I also thought he had been joking.

He looked disappointed at me, too, sighed and buzzed for the next patient.

He had, of course, been teasing her with his own particular dry sense of humour, which Edith appeared to enjoy, but also highlighted his assertion that he was 'different' to other GPs.

SHO Post 4 – Obstetrics

My final hospital posting was as an SHO in Obstetrics and Gynaecology. I was the most junior member of the team, which was led by the consultant, followed in order by senior registrar and registrar, then me. My role was to be first on call for the gynaecology wards and for most non-urgent problems on the labour and maternity wards. The midwives knew to contact the registrars for urgent issues in labour due to their greater experience and specific professional qualifications and skills. In addition, I would clerk patients into both units, and also see patients in gynaecology, antenatal and postnatal clinics, and assist in theatre. As you would expect, it was a very busy unit, even throughout the night.

I found obstetrics difficult and stressful especially, of course, around delivery time itself. Seldom in medicine, and life itself, is there an occasion in which there are such high hopes and expectations of a totally happy outcome, but with so many potentially sudden, unpleasant or even dangerous snags waiting to suddenly spoil things. Midwives have to deal with this all the time, and are skilled at helping to make childbirth as enjoyable and fulfilling an event as possible, under the circumstances.

There is a constant tension between midwives and obstetricians on the labour wards. The midwives are independent professional practitioners who manage most deliveries without any medical intervention; however, they need to call on the medics when labour goes wrong or progresses poorly.

As a junior doctor, I witnessed a lot of conflict between the two professions.

'Stay away from my ladies – they don't need doctors interfering in their childbirth,' was often said out loud, or was otherwise the unsaid undercurrent from midwives in their communications, particularly with the on-call registrars. I felt a slight confusion at this, as I seemed to spend a lot of time running around the labour wards seeing and treating the patients at the request of the midwives. Perhaps my opinion is a little skewed as I don't know how many 'normal' deliveries there were that did not require my input.

Most of my time was spent suturing episiotomies. Episiotomies are a gruesome-sounding procedure in which midwives perform a cut in a patient's perineum during childbirth. The cut is made, with local anaesthetic and scissors, into a posterior angle of the vagina, in order to widen the aperture to allow a baby to come out a bit more easily and to prevent a more nasty tear, which can cause far more problems than a neat cut.

Although midwives made the judgement about doing and performing the episiotomy, they were, in that hospital, not trained or allowed to suture them. Suturing these was the role of the SHOs, including me, and it often felt like I needed to suture one per hour throughout the night whenever I was on duty. The following year, the midwives were trained and expected to suture the episiotomies themselves. The percentage of deliveries needing episiotomies fell dramatically to half of what had been needed the year before.

The registrar on our team was Stavros, who was very helpful and hilarious in equal measure. On one occasion, we were waiting for the consultant, Mr Landis, in the sister's office before a ward round. Stavros was telling whoever would listen that his family had been reading *OK! Magazine* in their country and it contained an article stating that several members of our royal family were gay. We all laughed. He said we were all being fooled by a corrupt conspiracy between the press and the Queen, and that the truth would come out in time. We continued to argue with him.

Mr Landis came into the office at that point and spoke to me first, as I was nearest the door. 'What's going on in here? I could hear the ruckus halfway up the ward.'

I replied, 'Stavros was telling us that half the royal family is gay.'

Mr Landis responded quickly. 'It must the Greek blood in 'em. Come on, let's get on.'

Stavros shook his head but still managed to laugh as he followed us through the door and onto the ward.

Country Doctor

My twelve-month registrar placement was in a General Practice based in Uppermill, a small village on the edge of both the Pennines and the Peak District. I was lucky to get one of these twelve-month posts, because this practice was normally booked up years ahead for training. Somebody else had dropped out with a few months to go, giving me this great opportunity. I was especially pleased as I lived only a few miles away.

The area used to be in Yorkshire until the 1970s when the border was moved a few miles to bring it into Lancashire, becoming part of Greater Manchester a few years later. Some diehard survivors still display Yorkshire white rose flags in their gardens as an act of defiant pride. Most locals feel more connected with Lancashire, as they are closer to towns there than to Yorkshire ones. It is a pretty area, much greener than when the valleys were filled with working mills. Many locals have their roots and accents in the Pennine-mill past, although increasing numbers of 'comer-inners' work in Manchester and many have moved into gentrified barn and mill conversions. It was a great place to work and to live.

The surgery was an excellent practice, centred around one main practice building but also with a few branch surgeries in nearby villages. The practice had two training posts with two trainers and two trainees. My trainer was Dr Bill Wharton, a well-regarded and experienced GP. He had started the practice in the 1960s and remained very much the senior partner in every sense. He led the practice with a fairly light touch and his training support was of a similar style, which was generally more common in those days. He was planning to retire a few years later, hopeful of spending some time visiting his daughter, who lived in the USA.

My first day there began less smoothly than I had hoped. I was due to start at 9 a.m. but was still officially on call at my previous post till 8 a.m. The first of August was one of the big changeover days in the NHS, the other being 1st February (main changeover days are currently on the first Wednesdays of August and February). On these days, most junior hospital medical doctors moved to their next training post. My previous post until 8 a.m. was as an SHO in Obstetrics and Gynaecology. I had been on call the day and night before. This meant working nine till five and then overnight, covering the maternity and gynaecology wards as their first medical contact for routine and urgent issues on the wards. The duty registrar was based on the maternity wards for the more emergency calls.

On this particular changeover morning, the registrar had already left at 8 a.m., so I was left covering for the maternity and labour wards. I was checking a foetal-scalp blood gas sample for a baby in a delayed labour, just to ensure that all was well and basically to see if a caesarean section was needed or could be safely deferred a bit longer. This was not a test that I did very often, but I was apparently the only junior doctor available who had not yet escaped to their next job and the new intake had not started or even collected their bleeps or duty rotas yet. The baby was, thankfully, fine and I was safely able to leave the ward at 9.30 a.m. and collect my gear from my on-call room in the doctors' residence.

I had been working in that hospital for thirty months in a variety of junior and senior house officer posts. I walked through the grounds of the hospital to where my car was parked, stopping at the hospital switchboard to drop my bleep off. I vowed internally never to work in a hospital again. The exhaustion from another sleepless on-call night had obviously influenced that declaration, of course. I threw my overnight bag in the boot of my car and drove straight to the GP surgery. I arrived at 10.30 a.m., an hour and a half late. Not a great start.

'Glad You Could Make It'

Dr Wharton certainly did not appear very impressed with my punctuality, nor my excuses. He did, however, take me out on visits with him. He had come to work in his 1960s open-top white Mercedes Coupé.

It was a gorgeous hot sunny day and the visits were scattered around the lovely nearby villages and hills of Saddleworth. The contrast between my last hour of hospital work and my first hour in General Practice could not have been more dramatic. Life in General Practice looked like it was going to be much better than the past few years.

While my assumption turned out to be true, things were not always quite so rosy as they first appeared. It turned out that Dr Wharton usually only brought his Mercedes in on day one to impress and welcome trainees. It was a kind and thoughtful gesture nonetheless. The other part of his welcome routine that I remember from that first morning was a trip to one of the branch surgeries in another village. We parked up next to the surgery and I followed him on a short walk into a small local graveyard. Dr Wharton pointed out two particular family gravestones. They both told the sad stories of families devastated by the loss of young children: the first stone contained details of five children all dying in the 1870s, and all before they had reached eight years of age; the second showing the deaths of seven similarly young children in the 1820s. The assumption, and lesson, being that these children were most likely to have died from infectious diseases that we can now routinely vaccinate against, or at least treat effectively with antibiotics and other medicines. A sense of perspective and a reminder not to take things for granted and to recognise how lucky we were to have the benefits of such effective and life-saving treatments.

Bill dropped me back at main surgery so I could receive the induction to the practice that I had missed earlier from the practice manager. I also got chance to catch up with the other registrar, Mary, who I knew from our overlapping hospital posts. She was annoyingly brilliant at everything medical, and was also so friendly and compassionate that all patients, nurses and receptionists loved her, too. She and her GP husband, Bob, were a little eccentric and old-fashioned; both driving thirty-year-old classic cars and dressing within that same vintage. They were a good match for the surgery and its surrounds, which all seemed to belong to an altogether different era from the local hospital, five miles away, which I had just left for good.

(I recently drove back to the village to have a look at the gravestones mentioned previously, to check on the details, thirty-odd years after I last saw them. At first, I was a bit disorientated and could not see the stones where I remembered them. After a few minutes, I found them. They had both been moved and were now lying horizontal on the grass, heavily overgrown with moss. I scraped the moss off so that I could see and read the inscriptions. I suspect it won't be long till they are both overgrown again, probably forever this time, taking their sad stories from centuries past with them.)

Day Release

GP registrars spent one day a week in a training session at the local district general hospital. My trainer referred to the day-release course as playschool, in order to irritate the registrars: a tradition that I was delighted to continue with my registrars, years later, of course. Ten or so local trainees were taught GP skills by an experienced local GP, Rob Merton, who had a very gentle and relaxed teaching approach. His style being similar to the comedic actor Ronnie Corbett, lacking only a pipe, slippers and roaring log fire for a complete warm picture of cosiness. Like most good teachers, he allowed us to feel as if we had come up with the agenda and ideas every week as he led us gently to our conclusions, which seemed surprisingly similar to his by the finish.

We were taught that the chief concepts in successful GP consultations involve establishing what the *patients'* ideas, concerns and expectations were, with regard to their symptoms or illnesses – not the GPs, otherwise the time and effort of the whole consultation could be wasted. Any treatment plans should also be shared and agreed between the GP and the patient, as patients are far more likely to follow a plan that they understand and can see the point of.

It may seem a strange thing to have to learn how to conduct a consultation. It certainly may seem a bit alien, or at least a bit of a luxury. You may think that a GP consultation should be like that in A&E; the patient comes in, having had an accident or an illness, and shows or tells the doctor what their problems are, and the doctor treats the condition. That idea is OK in the emergency setting, but less so in General Practice.

An example of things going wrong was demonstrated many years later on reviewing videos of two consultations undertaken by a registrar based at the next-door practice, which he kindly shared with us. The consultations involved a mum bringing her young son to the GP on two separate occasions. At the first visit, it was revealed that the child had a cough. The trainee examined the boy, diagnosed a viral illness and suggested giving the boy paracetamol and fluids. The mum and boy came back three days later. The child still had a cough but was not unwell. The trainee listened to his chest again, then issued a prescription for an antibiotic and handed it to the mum.

She said, 'What's that?'

He replied, 'It's a prescription for an antibiotic.'

She said, 'I thought you said it was a viral infection.'

'I did. I do,' said the registrar.

'Then why have you given him an antibiotic?'

The registrar replied, 'Because I thought that's what you wanted.'

'Well, I don't.'

The registrar now looked perplexed and asked, 'What have you come back for, then?'

'I wanted you to listen to his chest to see if it's clear. His cousin is in hospital with pneumonia and I wanted to make sure he didn't have it.'

'You should have said,' said the doctor.

'You should have asked,' said the mum tartly, adding, 'Does he need an antibiotic then?'

'No,' said the chastened doctor.

'OK, thanks,' said the mum, standing up. She scrunched up the prescription and left it on the doctor's desk, saying, 'I won't be needing this.' She left, holding her son's hand.

It seemed likely that if the registrar had spent a bit longer at the initial consultation exploring the mum's concerns, then she may have not felt the need to come back for a second.

Many different consultation models have been put forward and studied in order to see what elements both good and bad consultations contain, in an effort to understand the dynamics and patterns contained therein. The overall idea being that registrars, and also experienced doctors, should use those successful structures and patterns to help guide consultations to be better and more focused on the patients' needs. There is also the need to be on the lookout for hidden agendas in the patient's presentation: these can be consciously or subconsciously hidden. They are less likely to remain hidden if the patient is allowed to feel comfortable enough to share, sometimes embarrassing, problems with the doctor.

It is very common for patients to leave the revelation of their most serious complaints until they stand up, hand on the door handle, ready to leave:

'Oh, yeah, just before I go – I've been coughing up blood.

A lot.

For a month.'

Another great benefit of the course was the opportunity to talk to all the other registrars working in different types of practice, with the bonus of a proper lunchtime thrown in. It turned out that hospital canteen food at lunchtime was actually quite nice. Who knew? I certainly didn't, as I seldom had the chance for a sit-down lunch when I was a house officer and only found out after I left my hospital posts. Another reason to appreciate the joys and relative freedom of our new life in General Practice.

Cat Woman

Yvonne was a lovely lady in her seventies who came to see me in the surgery in order to find out the results of a blood test, which had been arranged by one of the practice's previous registrars.

Yvonne had been suffering from an intermittent cough and wheeze. Her symptoms and signs were akin to asthma but had developed a bit later in life than usual, hence my predecessor had arranged a blood test to confirm his presumptive diagnosis of an allergy to cat fur. Yvonne had four cats. The blood tests confirmed that she had this allergy, specifically to cat fur. We discussed the result and implications of these results. As you would perhaps expect, she had no intention of getting rid of her beloved cats. She was also not keen on changing the living arrangements for the cats: she still intended that they should continue to sleep in her bedroom and to spend the daytime in the living room with her. This was not a big surprise to me. I have never known anybody with a pet allergy to want to give up having the pets, although sometimes room access has been adjusted appropriately.

Yvonne was keen for us to try to help her manage her symptoms when they were troublesome. She had already been using antihistamine tablets, with little benefit so far. I decided to prescribe an inhaler to help her. This was a salbutamol metered-dose inhaler – a typical blue-coloured inhaler that was frequently used for asthma and bronchitis patients at that time. These inhalers squirt out a fine mist containing the drug and are squirted into the mouth while inhaling before trying to hold one's breath for up to ten seconds. She seemed pleased that she had a potential treatment for her cat allergy.

A few weeks later, I spotted her name in the visit book following my morning surgery. She had apparently deteriorated and was even unable to come into the surgery to be seen. This was unusual for her. I wanted to see her so took this visit and grabbed her notes as well as a few others.

She lived a few miles away in a small, pretty stone cottage in the hills above a nearby village. She let me in. She was noticeably wheezy while walking back to her armchair. Two cats were sat on this chair and a few others close by. A quick examination confirmed the wheeze was present in both of her lungs. I was a bit perplexed and surprised that she was worse. I had not expected to cure her, but did hope for some small improvement at least. I considered adding another type of inhaler to her treatment regimen but then thought about a recent lecture on asthma that I had attended on the trainee day-release course. One of the key messages from this lecture was to check on patient compliance before stepping up treatments. This included inhaler technique: some patients did not coordinate the spray with their inhalation or did not hold their breath properly. I realised that I had not spoken to this lady about this, nor demonstrated it properly.

I asked her to show me how she was using the inhaler. She picked it up, pointed it at the nearest cat and squirted it at its face. The cat sneezed and shook its head. Yvonne continued to spray the inhaler at its back as it jumped off the chair. She pointed it another cat before I stopped her. I wanted to laugh but resisted: this lady was feeling ill and it was my fault, really, as I had failed to explain or show her how to use the inhaler.

We started again. She understood my belated instructions and had a little chuckle herself. The cats had all moved a bit further away and looked slightly wary until she put the inhaler down.

I saw Yvonne again for a review a few weeks later, this time back in the surgery. She had been a lot better, thankfully, and was happy to carry on with this type of inhaler. I trust that her cats were also able to relax a bit more again.

Wintersong

Just before Christmas, I was called to visit a young child suspected of having an ear infection. It took me a while to find the property as it had a name rather than a number and was way out in the countryside. It turned out to be a large converted barn, with nearby stables and paddock. A few horses were being led across the yard, so I drove past them slowly towards the barn and parked alongside a large 4x4. I got out and knocked on the large arched door. I was greeted by a smart bearded chap in his forties, who ushered me into the hallway and told me the story of his son's current illness and his concerns. He then led me past a large open living room, centred around a beautiful full-size grand piano. We went upstairs and along the landing towards his son's room. There were several gold discs hung on the wall.

I asked the fairly obvious. 'Are you a musician?'

'Yes,' he replied.

I didn't recognise him, so I asked, 'Are you a solo musician or in a group?'

'In a group.'

He then told me the group's name, which I did recognise.

'Oh, gosh,' I said.

'We're not very famous nowadays: not in Britain, anyway,' he said.

By that time we had arrived at his son's room. We went in and I spoke to and then examined his son. He did have an ear infection and obviously felt miserable with this. I left a script for a suitable antibiotic with his dad, who then showed me out, and we wished each other a happy Christmas.

I drove back towards the surgery for my evening surgery, remembering the one hit song by the band that I was familiar with. I remembered trying to play it on my guitar when I was in the sixth form at college. It was a kind of seasonal, if not fully Christmassy, song. It was then that I also remembered where I'd seen the dad's face before: on the front of a T-shirt worn by one of my college classmates, who was a big fan of the band. Another big fan turned out to be the Radio 2 DJ John Dunn, who played their hit song on his programme as I drove home later, after my evening surgery.

New Year Calling

Some of my GP friends like living in the area in which they work. They enjoy being the local GP and being well-known in their community. I prefer a degree of anonymity, having experienced living within the practice catchment area while I was a registrar. During that time, I was shouted at by a patient who was working behind the counter at the local sandwich shop.

'I'm a bit better, Doc; thanks for seeing me yesterday.'

This in front of a long queue in a full shop. I distinctly remembered his infected perianal abscess. My appetite for a sandwich suddenly vanished, even though I am sure he had washed his hands, so I ordered something pre-wrapped.

Although we are sworn to confidentiality, many patients don't appear to have the same shyness about sharing their ailments in a public place, often quite loudly. When Viagra was first launched, to much hype in the UK, I was frequently assailed in the local pub with loud requests for a prescription, often from men who had actually seen me in the surgery about this matter.

'Come on, Doc – gimme some Viagra.'

This was obviously less funny by the tenth occasion on the same night. Hard, then, to stop the other bar attendees from trying to have a quick word about their or their family members' health or delayed appointments or missed diagnoses.

On New Year's Eve during my registrar year, I was at home drinking with an old school chum. At midnight, the doorbell rang. It was a neighbour from the end of my road. He asked me to come and visit his wife, who was having a panic attack. I remembered his wife, as I had seen her in the surgery a few times with her anxiety problems. She was also under the care of the local community mental health team. Having established that she did not appear to be in any acute physical danger, I declined to visit, on the grounds of my high alcohol intake that evening. I suggested that he should ring the duty doctor service. The husband was not very happy and asked me again just to pop up and have a look. I was just about sober enough to assert that this was not a good idea and that he should ring the duty doctor service. He remained unhappy but left. I felt guilty, despite my belief that I had given the safest advice. Mick was irritated on my behalf and supported my decision, but our New Year celebrations were a little muted and foreshortened afterwards.

I saw this chap's wife in the surgery a few days later and she told me that she was OK now, but had just had an argument with her husband at New Year. He had not sought any other medical advice after speaking to me that night. I remained their neighbour for another year, but her husband never spoke to me again.

Cannibal

I was on a duty day and had left the surgery to do an urgent visit. On my return, one of the younger receptionists, Lisa, called me over. She looked a bit flustered.

She said, 'You've got another visit. Sorry. We were just about to bleep you.'

'It's OK,' I replied, trying to not look hacked off that my chances of a quick lunch seemed to be disappearing fast. I asked, 'What's the visit for?'

Lisa's face went a bit redder and she replied, 'Well ... it's some man, Mr Banks, who wants a visit for his son. He said he's a cannibal or something.'

One of the older receptionists, Brenda, chipped in then. 'He kept saying it was really important and that he wanted you to see his son, who's got a bad headache. He's six. Mr Banks seemed really odd and cocky. Apparently he told Lisa that he was a cannibal. Sorry.'

I paused a little after hearing this bizarre explanation of the visit request.

'That all sounds a bit weird. Do you think he was mad?' I asked.

Brenda screwed her face up and said, 'No, but he was full of himself, from what I heard.'

Lisa still looked embarrassed and just shook her head, then spoke again. 'Are you going, 'cos he was worried about his son?'

'I'll ring him back first. Have you got the number?'

Lisa shook her head again and said, 'No. They've just moved in and there's no phone connected yet. It's that new converted mill, past the branch surgery. Number 8. He rang from a phone box. Sorry.'

I drove up to and then through the next village, hoping the son was OK but also wondering what sort of person would describe himself as a cannibal. I parked up outside the mill, which was in the process of being renovated and still had lots of builders' and plumbers' vans outside. I went to the front door of number 8: a smart stone townhouse. Mr Banks, I presumed, let me in. He spoke and dressed loudly: wearing a red striped shirt, a blue tie and pink braces.

'Come in. He's upstairs. Sorry to drag you out, but I've got an important meeting in Manchester this afternoon. My wife's home later, though.'

We discussed his son's symptoms for a few minutes. He had been worried about the possibility of meningitis. We went up to see his son, who was feeling quite poorly and turned out to have tonsillitis. I issued a prescription for an antibiotic and discussed other supportive measures that his dad could do, and his mum, too, when she got home later. I went back downstairs to the kitchen, closely followed by Mr Banks.

He spoke again, 'Thanks for popping round. I would have brought him down to the surgery, but I've got a big interview to do this afternoon. I know your job is important, too, but y'know.'

I'd waited long enough. His son was not as ill as he and I had feared.

It was time to ask.

'What is that you do exactly? The receptionists seemed a bit confused.'

He puffed out his chest and said, 'I'm a headhunter.'

Ah. That explained it.

Not quite a cannibal, then, but I could see why Lisa had got confused. I had read about so-called headhunters in *The Sunday Times*. They recruited people for jobs, usually for big businesses or in the city. It was a relatively new term in the eighties and had come over from the States. Like Lisa, I had grown up hearing the term as description of certain tribes in Indonesia and perhaps South America. Maybe those headhunters were not all cannibals either, but were more likely to be so than a pompous recruiter in northern England was.

I was called to reception as soon as I arrived back at the surgery. Lisa, Brenda and the other receptionists were very keen to know what Mr Banks was on about. The truth was far less exciting than their speculations, so they soon lost interest.

My trainer, Bill, came into reception and said, 'Oh, you're still here. I thought you might be on display in some mud hut by now.'

I replied, 'Thanks for your touching levels of concern.'

I saw Mr Banks in the surgery a few times after that and he seemed all right, to be fair, apart from his habit of continually regaling the receptionists and other patients with tales from his important work.

Good Hair Day

One of my joint visits with Dr Wharton was to Mrs Croft, a smartly dressed eighty-year-old lady, who lived half a mile from the surgery. He generally visited her monthly to check her blood pressure and also her osteoarthritis. She was friendly and offered us both a cup of tea. We did not have time for that but thanked her for her kindness, of course. Dr Wharton arranged a follow-up visit and scribbled this in her notes.

A few weeks later, I was getting a lift with him to a post-graduate lecture at the local hospital. He pulled over to the side of the road shortly after leaving the surgery. Walking swiftly on the opposite pavement was Mrs Croft; no walking stick in sight.

Dr Wharton wound down his window and spoke. 'Hello, Barbara.'

'Hello, Dr Wharton,' she replied chirpily.

'Where are you going?' Dr Wharton asked.

'I'm going to the hairdressers,' she replied, slightly less chirpily now.

'But I'm due to visit you tomorrow,' stated Dr Wharton.

'I know. I always get my hair done for your visit,' she replied.

'Well, you don't need to bother from now on. You can come and see me in the surgery in future,' he said quite sternly. 'Starting tomorrow.'

She flushed a little and replied with a chastened, 'Yes, Dr Wharton.'

With that, he wound up the window and we drove off. We stopped at the main road, waiting to turn left when the traffic eased.

He turned to me and said, 'I know that I visit her for a chat as as much as medical reasons, but that's taking the mick.'

Home Visit

My trainer came back into the surgery reception after his visits. He looked stressed and a bit grey-faced.

He spoke to the practice manager and me at the same time. 'Norma, can you get me a coffee? Martin, will you come to my office?'

He walked straight to his room. Norma and I exchanged looks.

Norma said, 'Someone's in trouble. You'd better go through. I'll bring his coffee in and I'll get you one, too.'

I muttered my thanks and walked towards Dr Wharton's room, worried about what I must have done.

'Sit down,' he said as I went in.

'Is everything all right?' I asked with a forced grin.

'Not really,' he replied.

'Is it something I've done?' I asked.

'Oh, God, no,' he replied.

I breathed out through pursed lips, relieved.

'I have just been on the grimmest visit you could imagine. Remember that farmer I told you about? George Bradley? The one with lung cancer who lives up just past Hope Farm?' he asked.

I nodded and grunted my affirmation. Just then, Norma popped in with two coffees.

Dr Wharton said, 'Oh, you've brought Martin one, too. I'm not sure he's earnt it.' He winked at me as Norma exited, with her still wondering what I must have done, or not.

He continued, 'Well, I went to visit him 'cos he's refusing to have any treatment or even to go back to any hospital clinic again.'

'How is he doing?' I asked.

'Well, he's coughing up blood. Lots of it. He's spitting it out into a bucket in his kitchen.'

'That sounds awful. What are you going to do?' I asked.

He ignored my question and continued, 'That's not the worst of it. He had to lock the dog in the scullery 'cos it was going mad trying to get at the bucket. It was like a wild animal.'

'That is awful. I'm not surprised you wanted a coffee,' I said, while picturing the grotesque scene that was just described.

'And then,' he continued, 'the bloody dog burst in and stuck its head in the bucket, knocking it over. There was blood all over the floor and the dog, too. It was like a horror film. Shocking.'

'What did you do?' I asked.

'Well, I let him grab the dog and lock it up again. It was even trying to get at his face while he was shoving it back in the other room.'

'How is he going to manage?' I asked.

'Well, he's persuaded his brother to look after the dog and the brother is also cleaning up the kitchen for him. He's still refusing to go back to hospital or have any treatment. The danger is that that it [the cancer] will erode into an artery and he'll drown or die from blood loss. Not a nice way to go,' he said, and then, 'Will you visit him tomorrow, 'cos I'm not in?'

I could hardly say no but was not looking forward to that visit. In part because of the extreme grimness of it all and in part because I was not sure what more I could do to help him. I needn't have worried in that way; George was admitted to hospital during the night as his haemoptysis* had become more severe. While there, he later received some localised radiotherapy treatment to try to reduce the bleeding. Sadly, though, George remained an inpatient and continued to deteriorate until passing away just over a week later.

---

* Coughing up blood, or bloodstained mucous, from the lungs or throat.

A Grand Day Out

Towards the end of the GP training scheme, registrars had to take part in exams in order to be accepted as a GP. At that time, an additional option was also to take the Royal College of General Practitioner's (RCGP) exam so that you could add the letters MRCGP (Member of the RCGPs) after the other letters indicating your medical degrees. It held a certain kudos and was kind of expected if you wanted to apply for good jobs. I entered for this and scraped through the written part of the exam, so was invited to attend for the final oral (interview) part of the exam in London. This was to be completed at the RCGP headquarters at 14 Prince's Gate, near to the Albert Hall. This college building had become briefly more famous in 1980, as it was next door to the Iranian Embassy, the scene of the infamous siege in which six armed Iranians took twenty-six hostages. The siege ended when a team from the Special Air Service (SAS) entered the Embassy, having used the RCGP headquarters as their base. The Embassy was badly damaged by a fire during the siege.

I was on call at the surgery on the night before my exam but was allowed to finish my duties early at 11 p.m. instead of covering the whole night. I caught the 5 a.m. train from Manchester Piccadilly to Euston. It was a beautiful summer day in London so I decided to walk to Prince's Gate instead of taking the Tube. I remember passing Tower Records in Piccadilly Circus, hoping I would get the chance to call in on my way back later. I arrived at the college for 9.30 a.m. as requested, noting the scaffolding still covering the blackened Embassy next door, and queued up to look at the noticeboard, which had everyone's exam times posted on. Mine was at 4 p.m. Bloody hell.

I wished they would have released that information the day before so that I could have had a later, and more relaxed, journey. I wandered into Hyde Park to try to revise and to kill the six and a half hours of time before I was needed. I spent the whole time sat on a park bench in the lovely sunshine, half reading and idly half watching people playing tennis. I had a headache by my exam time, along with some sunburn, but managed the interviews OK. After that I walked back towards Euston, passing again through Piccadilly Circus, amazed to find Tower Records still open in the evening (remember – I was from the North and had also only been to London a few times before). I thought I had earnt a treat so spent half an hour buying a few LPs* I had been after for a while. An excellent result from a grand day out in London, and I got home for midnight.

I passed the exam, so I suppose that was an even better result.

In contrast, most of our current registrars take a few weeks' study leave off before any exams and will often stay over in London for a few nights to avoid travel fatigue. Different times, but to be fair, the current practical exam is much more onerous and time-consuming than ours was, although the college is now next door to Euston station so is a bit handier for doctors from the North West (and Tower Records is no longer there anyway!).

---

* Long Play or Long-Playing record. A 12-inch analogue sound storage medium with an album on; superseded by the CD. (A plastic disc containing digital information, such as recorded sound. Still purchased by many older music consumers but mostly superseded by digital downloads for the more digitally aware older consumers, or by streaming by younger consumers or ultra-trendy older consumers.)

Proper Job

I was twenty-seven when I became a GP partner. The advert for the vacancy had appeared in the *British Medical Journal* towards the end of my GP registrar placement year. At that time, there was quite a lot of competition to get a lifetime (hopefully) post in a partnership. I was very pleased to get this job in a good practice, in Ashton-under-Lyne, only five miles away from where I was living at that time. This felt like just about the perfect distance out for me, as I didn't really want to live within the practice catchment area, nor be too far out, particularly for the on-call visits. I was told later that there had been over a hundred applicants, but I had been shortlisted as I lived nearby and my trainer had given me a good verbal reference. The GP partners were all welcoming and friendly at my interview – the partners being four men and two women; three of the men were in their fifties, one in his forties and the two female partners in their thirties. I was helped in the interview by my local knowledge garnered in part from my on-call experience covering the practice area. I received the job offer later via phone call that same night. I felt very lucky.

The terms at that time were to be a salaried partner for twelve months and if I stayed, to then work up to a full share of GP income after three years. That was the norm at that time, but nowadays new GP partners would be expected to be paid a full share immediately or very soon after a brief introductory period. When I started out, GP jobs were scarce and it seemed like a great honour to be accepted into the club. Things have switched around completely now, as it is very hard to get good recruits who want to commit themselves to a lifetime at the same practice, especially as a business partner, and even more so as full-time.

Some of my friends and peers applying for jobs at that time still had to undergo 'trial by sherry', in which their wives also needed to meet the partners' wives in a social setting to make a decision on whether they were the 'right sort', too. Very old-fashioned and misogynistic even in those times. Fortunately, many of those boys'-club rules and barriers had already been broken down before my arrival, by the presence of female partners. Other friends told me that golf club membership had been heavily encouraged and interviews concluded on the course. Imagine the difficulties approaching that sort of practice as a female or gay person (or both), especially if you didn't play golf. You might not want to work in that type of practice, of course, but opportunities were quite limited.

I completed my training post on Monday, 31st July 1989 and started in my proper job as a real GP the following day.

Fine Dining

When on call, we used to have a Saturday morning surgery for urgent cases. After the surgery, the duty GP would be on call for visits until late evening and then again on the following Sunday from 7 a.m. We took this in turns, as well as sharing the evening duties during the week. We also covered for the other GP practice based in our health centre and they covered for us, although less frequently, as they had fewer patients and GPs.

On my very first Saturday morning surgery, I saw a lady who had requested an appointment as she had abdominal pain. I walked from my room to the waiting room and shouted her name. She followed me into the room and sat down. She was in her mid-forties and winced in discomfort as she sat down. She told me that she had been suffering from stomach pains all night and on further questioning, also admitted to having had a few bouts of diarrhoea. This was sounding like gastroenteritis of some sort. I asked if she had eaten anything unusual or 'dodgy'.

She sighed and looked a bit guilty. 'I had a Chinese last night.'

She agreed that her upset tummy was likely to be related to something in that meal. Nobody else in the household was poorly but nobody had ordered the same food as she had. She still looked uncomfortable and was still wincing occasionally as she spoke.

I suggested that I examined her, just to make sure I wasn't missing anything else. Her temperature was slightly raised, which fitted in with the presumptive diagnosis. I asked her to lie on the examination couch. She pointed to the area of most pain – this was in her epigastrium (the upper, central part of her abdomen, just under the ribs). I pressed there fairly gently and she was obviously quite tender. I asked if she had had this type of pain before.

'Yes, about five years ago.'

'What happened?' I asked.

'I had a Bavarian meal.'

That caught my attention, as do most references to food. I had once been for a Bavarian meal at a restaurant in the nearby Peak District and was very happy to hear of another.

'Where was that?' I asked.

She frowned and looked at me, confused.

'At the hospital, of course.'

After a few moments the penny dropped.

'Do you mean a barium meal?' I tried.

'Yeah, that's it.'

A barium meal was an X-ray examination after having a drink containing barium. This shows up clearly on X-rays so was used to try to outline the oesophagus, stomach and duodenum. It was a test used to look for ulcers, among other things. This meant that she was previously investigated for suspected peptic ulcer disease.

We decided to treat this current flare-up of pain and diarrhoea as gastroenteritis, but to book another appointment if her symptoms did not resolve soon.

She left wondering, I think, whether the new GP was properly qualified. I was left slightly disappointed that I had not discovered a new restaurant to try.

Finer Dining

New partners in General Practice could still feel a bit isolated at first but in my area had the benefits of a 'Young Principals' group, who met monthly in our local hospital post-graduate department for a chat and mutual support. This was sometimes followed by a trip to the pub. Some of the Young Principals were a bit older than you might expect and there was no formal cut-off age for being a member. Our club died out after a year or so when we were no longer allowed evening access to the department and actually, having the entire meeting in a pub did not sit right. We met for a few meals out, but most people drifted away as they married and had children or took on more evening duties.

I was fortunate enough to stay in touch with some of the doctors from my training practice and also from the one I had spent some study leave in, which included Dr Astley's partner, Dr Austin. They had their own informal meals out every few weeks or so, often sponsored by 'drug reps', these being pharmaceutical salespeople whose job was to sell their products to hospitals and GPs. They often had generous budgets and were keen to support social gatherings, often with minimal actual product advertising done, beyond the mention of the drug's name. Dr Austin was very sociable and would arrange many of the meals out. Like me, he hated snobbery and pomposity, but was a bit more direct than I was at trying to puncture it.

Our dining club gave us the chance to eat at some smart restaurants beyond our income at the time, including one with a French name near to Manchester Airport. There, I made the mistake of asking for a glass of beer before my meal, only for the waiter to give an audible gasp before he then sniffed at me.

'This is a fine dining establishment, sir, not a pub. We don't serve beer.'

Despite his sniffiness, we still behaved ourselves and enjoyed the food, if not his attitude and overall atmosphere.

A few weeks later we were fortunate enough to be entertained at the French Room restaurant in the famous Midland Hotel in Manchester. This being the legendary meeting place of Mr Rolls and Mr Royce and also, apparently, a favourite haunt of Winston Churchill whenever he was in town. Dr Austin decided to test the snobbery of the waiters there, in comparison to those in the snooty airport restaurant.

'Red or white?' asked the wine waiter as he stood poised by the table, a bottle in each hand.

Dr Austin looked at me first, with raised eyebrows, then replied to the waiter, 'Half of each, in the same glass, please.'

The waiter did not blink. He poured both wines at the same time while maintaining full eye contact with Dr Austin.

'Certainly, sir. You know best,' he replied, without any audible trace of sarcasm. He finished his round of the table, completely professional and unflappable.

Dr Austin sipped his wine after the waiter left, saying, 'This is disgusting, but I'd better drink it now.'

On another occasion, Patrick (Dr Austin) had invited his close friend, Carl, along with us for a meal. Carl was a shopkeeper, but Patrick had told him that if he pretended to be a GP then he would get a free meal, courtesy of the drug rep. Patrick promised Carl that he and I would help him to deal with any questions so that he would not be found out. On the night, the rep and other doctors spent most of the time questioning Carl. We helped him out but it was apparent that Carl was a bit uncomfortable: flushed and sweating and not eating much at all. As we finished the meal, Patrick told Carl that the other doctors and the rep all knew his secret all along. It was all a bit mean but seemed funny at the time, at least for the rest of us. Carl relaxed a bit more after the revelation and ordered more food, as his appetite picked up a bit when his anxiety cooled down.

The opportunities for this type of sponsored meal declined over the next few years as advertising rules were tightened. For many years now the reps have not even been allowed to gift GPs or hospital doctors with so much as a cheap pen or sticky pad, as this is now seen as bribery. Perhaps so, and apparently fair enough, but these dinners allowed time for valuable depressurising and mutual support, and also allowed some good friendships to develop between doctors and also many of the reps. My wife, Michelle, is a medical rep who I first met thirty years ago. Our paths crossed again ten years ago, at first professionally and then socially; the rest is our history, at least.

Fit as a Doctor's Dog

The first time I was offered a glass of whisky on a home visit was at 11 a.m. on a wet February day. I declined.

'Dr Lang always has one when he visits,' said the patient. Dr Lang had retired recently.

The second time, on another day, visiting another patient, I was offered a double whisky, on this occasion at 10.30 a.m. I again declined.

The patient's husband said, 'Dr Lang used to always have a whisky. We liked him. He was one of us.'

I apologised for my apparent ingratitude and thanked them for their kindness.

'I never drink in the daytime and certainly never when I am at work or driving.'

'Well, Dr Lang seemed to manage OK and everyone liked him,' said the patient herself, resentfully.

Despite my wish to be liked, I continued to find the strength to refuse.

I was offered whisky on numerous other occasions while visiting, often as soon as I had walked through the front door. On every occasion I refused and on every occasion I was referred to the warm-hearted acceptance of such kindness by my beloved predecessor.

Other patients told me how they used to bump into Dr Lang in their local pub, where he stopped by for 'a few pints and a whisky chaser' while he was out walking his dog. I soon worked out that he would call at one pub at 7 p.m. and another at 7.30 p.m. and another at 8 p.m., and perhaps more after that. He and his pooch obviously walked a bit further each night than most of the patients realised. The dog was probably quite fit – or at least a bit healthier than Dr Lang's liver.

I was not aware of this complete drinking pattern during the brief time that we were both working at the same practice. The partners knew that he 'liked a drink', but not perhaps quite how much, or how often.

One of his neighbours latterly revealed that he had discovered Dr Lang stashing alcohol bottles in trees and bushes along his dog-walking route. The neighbour had often collected and thrown away these bottles, as he was so disgusted at this behaviour.

Many of his patients seemed to retain fond memories of Dr Lang and I don't recall ever hearing any of them complain about him or his treatment of them or their families, which was not automatically the case for all of the previously retired partners. They seemed very fond of him and his kindness, and many of them appeared to have liked the fact that he had this foible, which perhaps marked him as human, like them. Like the doctors, though, they are unlikely to have known the full extent of his problems, and the potential danger that put him and them in.

Military Tattoos

I'd been working at the practice for twelve months when my predecessor rang to tell me that he was passing on one of his outside job roles to me. He'd been working as a doctor for the local Territorial Army (TA) unit. This involved attending the unit every Wednesday night for three hours. I was not given the option of refusing as it was regarded as an honour, and there was a modest fee attached. My role was to conduct medical examinations for new recruits to the TA and to review the records of ex-soldiers who transferred from active to reserve duties. As you might expect, there was also a great deal of confusing Ministry of Defence (MOD) paperwork, which took a while to get to grips with.

The recruits were mostly new to the military, although a few army veterans came through into the reserves. After the initial medical examination, one of the requirements was to record the position of and description of their tattoos. Every recruit seemed to have quite a few and seemed happy to have them recorded. They were very proud of this expression of their individuality and a bit surprised that the MOD respected and required such accurate records. The reality was that these records were kept in order to try to identify bodies or body parts in any future conflict. I suppose that the recruits understood what they had signed up for and their potential fate.

One young recruit had seven tattoos on his arms – four on the right side, three on the left. All were different girls' names, so I asked him why.

He pointed to the name on his right upper arm.

'She said she'd shag me if I had her name tattooed on my arm, so I did, and she did. All of the others said the same thing when they saw the other names.'

It was a kind of foreplay, I suppose.

We both, at the same time, looked at the blank space on his left forearm.

'You might want to get a Velcro strip sewn in there.'

He smiled weakly and said, 'I had thought about transfers.'

I'm not sure that either of our proposed solutions would have met with MOD approval.

Practise in Practice

During the five years at medical school, and also in the first years working as a doctor, you are constantly being asked about what career path you plan on pursuing: also being reminded that a medical degree on its own does not give you a proper career, as further specialist training is still required. For the majority of us, a career in General Practice was expected and planned. I was in this majority: thinking I wanted a GP career, as I didn't know much about other specialities or choices, especially at the beginning. I tried to be open-minded to other options, but nothing else really tempted me away in the end. I suppose that working in A&E was the only other speciality that came close for me, but that lacked continuity.

One of the great things about General Practice is the opportunity to get to know patients over a longer period than is common in many other specialities. In my case, it also helps that I generally and genuinely am interested in people (being nosey), especially patients, and I enjoyed the friendship that develops with them and their families over the years. Not all patients, and not all of the time, of course, as you may be able to tell from the rest of my musings. We all have times in which we complain about our work and our workload, and the examples we tend to use to illustrate this are often at the more extreme end of this.

The majority of patients don't like to be a nuisance or to trouble doctors unnecessarily. Many downplay their symptoms. Most are more worried about their family than themselves. Even those who are struggling often surprise you when push comes to shove. Some patients who have appeared anxious or fragile during everyday life suddenly seem to develop tremendous resources and bravery when they fall seriously ill.

It has been a privilege to see and be able to help people when they really need it, and the relationship formed with them over the years often helps them to trust you at the most fragile times. Sometimes the relationship only fully develops during times of serious need; these patients or their relatives are often very loyal afterwards and try to see you whenever they or their families need help again.

Humour often seems to come at seemingly inappropriate moments and certainly gallows humour is very common in practice, and seems even more so in Northern patients. This often seems to help people cope with overwhelming stress. A GP needs to be very careful of jesting at delicate times but, obviously, a patient's filter and humour is allowed to be set a little more coarsely. One of my friends was a GP in North Manchester and had slightly misjudged the humour situation while talking to a patient's son. He was later featured on the front page of the *Daily Mirror* with the headline, 'GP in Sell-by Shocker', after he had said to the chap:

'Let's face it, your mum's a bit past her sell-by date.'

I have never used that particular phrase with a patient, although I have heard it used it a good deal by patients themselves and also by their families. I was not afraid of teasing or joking with patients, but usually only after the patient had opened up that particular communication channel.

The Change

'Doctor. I'm really sorry to bother you, but can you please do me a massive favour?'

I looked up from my work computer and, more importantly, my sandwich, to see Anne, the nurse for the other GP practice with whom we shared a health centre. She was standing in the doorway and looked quite anxious.

'Of course. What is it?' I replied, trying to sound more enthusiastic than I felt.

'I've got this lady with me who's in a right state and none of our doctors are due back in till four.'

I looked at my watch. It was one o'clock.

Anne must have sensed my reluctance.

'She has been put on my list as an emergency. She's really upset and thinks she's got cancer.'

I sighed and stood up, putting my sandwich on the desk, after deciding it was impolite to keep Anne and her patient waiting.

'Oh, thanks,' she said. 'I've put her in the clinic room.'

The patient, aged fifty-six, thought that something, probably cervical cancer, was 'rotting down below'. She told me that the lady was on a trolley and had removed her skirt and underwear. I followed Anne to the clinic room and in we went.

'Hi, Kate,' Anne said. 'I've brought that nice doctor with me; he'll have a quick look for you.'

I introduced myself a bit more formally and asked Kate a few questions, confirming the brief history that Anne had given me. Things had apparently come to a head over the weekend as *Casualty*, on BBC One, had featured a patient with cervical cancer, but, more worryingly, the smell was becoming worse. I must admit that there was a bit of a nasty odour already in the clinic room. I wondered if somebody had been in earlier having a leg ulcer dressed. Anne held Kate's hand as I started my examination with the speculum.*

The smell had become overwhelming at that point and I wondered if it was possible for me to breathe through my ears. Alas, not. There was definitely a lump of sorts high up in this lady's vagina, just behind her cervix. I used some forceps and had a quick prod of the lump, which moved a little. I realised that it was a foreign body of sorts, so grabbed it and pulled it out with the forceps. It came out fairly easily after some initial reluctance and it turned out to be a slimy dark-grey tampon.

Anne looked queasy. I threw the offensive lump into the clinical-waste bin and explained to Kate, and Anne, what it was. I reassured her that she did not have any signs at all of cancer, hoping that she might be relieved. Instead, a look of confusion appeared on her face.

She frowned and said, 'But I don't use tampons.'

'Well, it was definitely a tampon,' I replied.

'But I'm on the change.'

'When did you last have a period?' I asked.

'Over two years ago.'

Well, it must have been there for two years, then, at least,' I said.

'I don't think so,' she said a bit shirtily. 'Can you both go out now, while I get changed.'

We did, with some relief, glad to breathe some fresher air. Kate rushed past us twenty seconds later, looking angry but more likely embarrassed.

Anne said, 'I don't know how I did not throw up in there. God knows how you managed.'

---

* The usually cold metal device used to allow vaginal examinations and smear tests.

I wasn't sure, either.

She added, 'How come she had that there for so long when some girls get toxic shock* after a day or two?'

A good question, for which I had no answer.

Anne nipped back into the clinic room to retrieve and double- and then triple-bag the offending article. This did not seem to help very much. I was unable to finish my sandwich so that, too, was binned and I went for a short walk instead, to clear my head and nostrils.

Days later, there was still quite an odour present throughout the health centre, long after the bins had been emptied. No wonder that poor lady had been so worried and embarrassed. She had also been incredibly lucky not to have developed a significant, even fatal, infection.

---

* Toxic shock syndrome is a potentially fatal condition caused by bacterial release of toxins, often associated with and caused by a tampon being left in place for longer than advised.

Next Door

It was a busy Sunday on-call day. By 10 a.m. I had received five visit requests from the answering service. The first request was to see an elderly lady who was known to have dementia, and who had become distressed and agitated during the night. Her husband had requested the visit as he didn't know what to do. I decided to call there first. I parked up outside the house, walked to the front door and rang the bell. The gentleman answering the door looked vaguely familiar to me and, indeed, recognised me, too.

'Oh, it's Dr S, isn't it?' he said.

'Yes.'

'I've seen you around in the surgery, but not had an appointment with you myself. Come in.'

He showed me into the back room and asked me to sit down. He also offered me a cup of tea, which I declined.

'How is your wife?' I asked.

'She's just getting up. She likes a bit more of a lie-in than I do. She'll be down in a minute.'

I was a bit surprised at how quiet the house was and how relaxed he looked under the circumstances. His wife came downstairs and into the living room.

'Dr S is here, love,' he said. His wife was dressed and looked smart, but also looked wary and confused.

'Oh, hello,' she said, while giving a sideways glance at her husband.

'Would you like a brew, love?' he asked her. She also declined and sat down, still looking at me warily.

Neither of them looked very distressed or upset. I thought I'd better get to the point, so directed a question to her.

'How have you been?'

'I'm OK, thanks.'

Time to ask the husband: 'Have things been difficult for you both?'

'Not really. Money can be a bit tight, but it's the same for everybody, isn't it?' he replied.

A tough crowd. I tried again, to the wife. 'Have you been anxious or upset recently?'

She shook her head. Lips pursed.

'Did you sleep OK? You've not been up all night?'

The husband chipped in again at this point. 'Well, we both got woken up last night by 'er, next door, didn't we, love? She's got dementia. Can't help it, poor thing, but it's not right. I don't know how her husband copes.'

Ah.

'What's your name?' I asked, a little belatedly.

'Knowles. We're Jack and Linda,' he replied.

Wrong house.

I confessed the mistake and that I had been given the wrong address. Linda looked a little happier and her husband continued in his usual avuncular manner.

He said, 'I thought it might be 'er, next door, that you wanted.'

I wondered to myself why he hadn't mentioned this earlier, but I was not really in a position to throw any blame, given that I had turned up at the wrong house and he had still welcomed me in. I thanked them both and he wished me good luck next door. His wife just shook her head at this stage, presumably at my incompetence. I went next door.

The lady with dementia who had been up all night was sleeping when I got there. Her husband had forgotten to give her her night-time sedatives until 4 a.m., then she had taken them and fallen quickly asleep. These days we don't recommend using medications such as these as they can increase daytime confusion and the risk of falls. The lady woke up while I was there and seemed calm, if still a little tired. She was due a follow-up visit on the Monday by her community psychiatric nurse, so I left. I walked back to my car and waved to the Knowleses, who were both already waving at me vigorously from their front window.

Weight for the Doctor

Throughout my first few years in General Practice, in the early 1990s, I often did locum sessions at other surgeries during my annual leave. I usually did these as a favour to GP friends or colleagues who were desperate to go away on holiday, but also to earn a bit of extra money, of course. It was always good to see how some of the other surgeries functioned and to pick up any good ideas or processes to take back to ours. One such idea was having one of the GPs spend the full morning doing visits, rather than the traditional scramble of all the doctors visiting after their morning surgery. This was especially useful if somebody sounded ill enough to need an early visit.

Some of these surgeries were in run-down premises in much more deprived areas than my own. One particular surgery in my home city of Salford had a very vague GP timetable, with management and reception staff unclear about when any of the doctors might be returning from extended holidays or family visits. This appeared to be the norm for them. I was surprised how relaxed the patients seemed to be about the very irregular and vague service they received. They appeared very grateful for the minimal interventions and support offered by the surgery, which made me realise that people will often put up with poor-quality and disrespectful care if that's all that seems to be available.

This was a massive contrast with my own surgery, which was well organised and with all the GPs, by then, working full-time in the practice only. We were all very supportive to our colleagues but also a bit more uptight with each other, if anyone was as much as a half-hour late for work. Our patients also seemed to have much higher expectations and demands from our practice. We offered vastly more GP and nurse appointments than any of the neighbouring surgeries and yet the demand was for even more. I suppose that our expectations of ourselves were also high and we tried to accommodate where possible, but even our resources and energies still had limits.

Some aspects of practice remained universal: patients could still be as baffling and amusing here as at any other surgery. At one morning surgery in the inner-city practice in Salford, my consecutive patients were identical red-headed twins in their late teens. They were dressed identically, too. If I had not already seen them together in the waiting room, I may have thought that the same patient had come back in as a joke. I shouted out the first name on my patient list at the consulting room door, and Twin One came in and sat down. She cut straight to the chase.

'Dr Fogerty put me on this new pill, Femodene, and I'm putting a load o' weight on with it. Can I change it, please?'

We discussed the reasons why she had changed to this contraceptive pill and other potential side effects with the likely alternatives. She was satisfied with my description of the one I now prescribed and left, happily clutching the prescription for the different breed and brand of pill. She stopped at the door and turned back to me, saying:

'Should I send our kid in?'

I thanked her but said that I would call her in soon, after I had written in the notes and worked out how to use the computer, which was working on a different system to the one I was most familiar with. Five minutes and ten swear words later, I called in Twin Two, although using her real name, of course. She sat down and was equally to the point as her sister.

'Dr Fogerty put me on this new pill, Femodene, and I'm losing a load o' weight with it. Can I change it, please?'

Slightly on the back foot, I muttered, 'Err, some people feel that they put weight on with this and other pills. Weight loss isn't that common.'

Of course, she and Twin One were free to speak to each other about their health concerns, but I was bound by confidentiality not to share details of their consultations. I discussed the alternative pills that were available, including the most likely potential side effects, of course. She picked the same one as her sister.

I would have liked to see how they both got on. A shame that I was not doing another locum at that surgery for their planned follow-up appointments in three months, or sooner. Most likely their individual weights would have carried on their divergent paths and they may have each requested yet another different pill.

On Call

One of the GP's statutory responsibilities was providing 24-hour cover for their patients, 365 days a year. When I was a registrar in my training practice, I was responsible for covering one weekday night from the surgery closing at 6 p.m. till opening the next morning at 8 a.m., as well as one full weekend in five. This was for our practice patients plus another local practice, on top of the normal working week. Although this appears to be quite onerous, it was so much less than the hospital working hours as to feel almost like part-time work.

When I moved into partnership the following year, the out-of-hours responsibilities remained, but the practice policy was to pay a local GP co-operative visiting service to cover our patients from 11 p.m. through till 7 a.m. on weekdays, so at least there was the opportunity to get a proper sleep. At weekends, the duty GP did a Saturday morning surgery followed by visits until late evening, when the visits were 'put through' to the co-op service until 7 a.m. on the Sunday: then it was back on duty for visits until 6 p.m. again.

Some of those days and nights could be really busy and a lot of time was spent driving from visit to visit across the wide practice area. Before mobile phones were widely available, we were bleeped by our answering service and then required to look for a working phone box, armed with a bagful of coins, in order to retrieve the visit request details. The bleep often went off a few times while you were still looking for a working phone.

One Christmas Day in the middle of the flu season, I was called to do fifteen visits in the morning alone and collected another two or three new visit requests by the time I got to the phone each time. I didn't mind working on that day and neither did I have any children at that time, which made things a little easier. I felt quite noble driving off my estate while everybody else was still getting up and unwrapping presents. I also knew I just had to get through this one day and I would have Boxing Day off. One other clear memory of this particular day was that the only two patients to thank me for visiting them were the two who were most seriously ill, one of whom I admitted to hospital (with pneumonia). No other patient or their relatives even mentioned the nature of the day, even while I was wading through piles of discarded wrapping paper to get to the patients' beds or sofas.

Many of the visits we undertook were for serious or worrying symptoms, although there was an increasing amount of less urgent problems as the years went by. Partly this was due to changes in expectations about health and suffering, compared to our parents and grandparents who tried to avoid troubling the NHS, often putting off accessing care much longer than they should. There was, however, a significant cohort of patients who rang at night as they would be seen at home quickly and without having to convince a receptionist of the urgency of their condition. There was also an inherent anonymity in calling the answering service, which was often then punctured by the appearance of their own GP at the door.

I was once called out late on a Saturday night to treat a lady for thrush, although the visit had been requested for an 'inability to walk'.

My colleague, Patrick, was called at 4 a.m. for a visit request by a female patient. His practice was semi-rural and they were expected to provide cover themselves through the night, as they usually had very few calls. He rang back.

A man answered and said, 'Hi, Doctor. I wonder if you could come and do a visit?'

'What is the problem?'

'Err. We've lost a condom.'

'Can you not just find it and pull it out yourselves?'

'No, we've tried.'

'Well, that is not urgent. Ask your wife to come to the surgery at nine o'clock and I'll fish it out.'

'Can you not come out now?'

'No, it's not an emergency,' said Patrick, increasingly irate.

'You don't understand. It's the only one we've got.'

That last cry for help did not incline Patrick any more to visit.

The lady did come to the surgery as requested, to have the condom removed by the now grumpy GP.

She spoke to him as he used a speculum and forceps to retrieve the item in question.

'Sorry about the phone call; I told him not to ring at that time, but he was a bit keen to go again.'

Out-of-hours cover by GPs was becoming an increasing problem, especially for more rural GP practices. In those areas, there were often not enough GPs available to provide any co-operative cover, which meant that GPs had to provide all of this cover: even more tiring if they were single-handed. This system was not so problematic in the 1940s and 1950s, when NHS General Practice was first established, but patient demand had changed over the years and the number of out-of-hours visit requests was increasing. Rural GPs in particular were affected by this, as they could also not easily get any locum cover for holidays.

The government, thankfully, responded to the situation by amending the GP contract so that GPs in England could opt out of this twenty-four/seven responsibility. The government kept back the six per cent of GP income dedicated to this portion of GP work in order to fund the changes and the replacement service. It did not take long until the true level of demand and cost were uncovered and the government considered holding back more money.

The changes to the system were heavily criticised by some elements of the press, who pursued the 'lazy GPs' narrative. It didn't help that GPs were given a pay rise at the same time, although this came with changes in the NHS GP pension system. These meant for most GPs, who are effectively self-employed, their pension payments rose from fourteen per cent of their gross income, up to twenty-nine per cent. The NHS had stopped paying the employer's portion of GPs' pensions. This high rate was paid only by higher earners and also included some monies to be paid into lower earners' pension pots. It turned out that the pay rise was more than swallowed up by the pension changes.

The NHS GP pension was still a good pension scheme to be in, but unlike many other parts of the NHS and other government pension schemes, was overpaid by its members: the amount paid in being higher than that taken out. At the time it did feel like another tax to be paid, but in the long run it allowed for a decent amount to be squirrelled away into the retirement pot.

Ben and Betty

Ben was a lovely and engaging man, in his late eighties when I first met him. He was of Chinese ancestry and he told me that his family had a local laundry business, which he also worked in as a little lad. Apparently, this was a common profession for Chinese immigrants before the British developed a taste for Chinese food. Ben had requested a visit for his wife, Betty, who was also, as you might expect, lovely. Sadly, though, she had developed some symptoms suggestive of dementia and Ben had reluctantly had to call us for help. He had been struggling to look after her and protect her from the consequences of her illness. They had a very supportive family too, but he and Betty were still very much a close couple, evidently still both wrapped up in each other's love.

Betty struggled at first to accept outside help from me and then the psychiatric and dementia support teams. Ben was very kind and patient with her and always able to talk her round to accepting support, even towards the end when she had deteriorated and taken to her bed. I always looked forward to my visits there, despite the sadness of Betty's inevitable decline, and I left with my spirits lifted by their humour and evident love for each other. Betty passed away at home, surrounded by her family.

A few months after her passing, some members of the family saw me on their own appointments at the surgery and expressed concern for Ben's future. They worried that he would struggle without Betty; in his case, his genuine other half. I called to see him, ostensibly to check on his welfare, but just as much for a chat and a catch-up. He seemed to be managing quite well, surrounded by photos and memories. He took me upstairs to see their bedroom and showed me that Betty's dressing table was still laid out as before. I noticed there was still a strong smell of perfume in the bedroom and pointed this out. Ben chuckled and produced a bottle of Chanel perfume from a drawer in the dressing table. He opened the wardrobe door and squirted the perfume on Betty's clothes, still hanging there.

'I do this every day. It was her favourite perfume and it means she's still here with me,' he said.

We went back downstairs and he told me that he had loved her since he first met her, in the 1930s. He told me how they, like many couples, had been separated during the war, initially when he'd left on basic training with the army. He told me about his thoughts when he had been on the train travelling to and from the barracks for the training or back home on leave. He told me that he sang a song in his head to the rat-a-tat of the train line: singing 'further away, further away' all the way out, and 'nearer to you, nearer to you' all the way back home.

Later on, he was sent overseas to war, to North Africa. He shivered when he told me about the Battle of El Alamein, and how the nearby guns had pounded constantly and loudly for many days. He said that he was so frightened by the noise and violence and just longed to get back home safely. He also stated that he was not brave, and that he was just a little Chinaman missing home and his beloved Betty.

I visited Ben a few times over the next few years: more frequently, sadly, after Ben developed lung cancer. He remained upbeat and chuckling even towards the very end, also often surrounded by his family. I still saw some of them in the surgery up until a few years ago. His daughter and granddaughter always asked me if I remembered Betty and Ben. Of course. It would be harder to forget them.

Expressions

I love the variety of language, especially local expressions and dialect. Living and working on the overlapping margins of Greater Manchester and Lancashire means exposure to phrases from both areas. Surprising to me when I started in the practice were the number of phrases I had never heard of, despite being born and raised only about ten miles away.

If you want to start an argument in the North, especially, just try describing a small fist-sized individual piece of bread to somebody. These appear to have a different name every few miles and people get very angry at the temerity of anybody else describing their lump of bread by the wrong name, or by how much they differ in thickness or flouriness to the neighbouring breads. The list includes – muffins, oven-bottom muffins, breadcakes, barm cakes, barms, bread rolls, rolls, stottie cakes, stotty and tufty buns. Many other names are available. If your bread lump of choice is not listed above, please try not to be too offended or angry or actually shout at the page.

A local phrase from patients, which completely threw me for a while, was 'I'm starved.' I initially asked patients if they had not had time to eat, but just got funny looks back and no sensible replies. I later found out that 'starved' meant 'freezing cold' rather than hungry.

Another common expression is 'rum', which is widely used as an adjective to describe somebody, usually a man who is odd or strange. In the North, the term is often even more ambiguous and is used to criticise somebody, but with an added hint of admiration; often describing a low-grade criminal or a chancer, although a 'rum 'un' can be anyone from a naughty child or an amusing local villain, up to and including a serial killer or dictator. For example, and in context, 'Ooh, that Vlad the Impaler was a right rum 'un.'

Another phrase that was sometimes used in normal everyday speech, but more frequently used by patients describing their medical encounters, is 'turned around', as in: 'He turned around and said to me.'

This was usually followed by: 'And I turned round to him and said ...' ad infinitum.

After many years of hearing this, I still find it hard to resist a secret smile at the thought of lots of people spinning around while talking to each other, in the manner of a whirling dervishes' convention.

'Rushed' is another common adjective. It is the only adjective ever used by patients to describe their, or their families', journeys to hospital.

As in, 'Mi dad was rushed into hospital with his leg last night.'

Very often, I've been the GP who'd admitted the patient referred to, and in virtually every case there was no rushing involved. The dad in the above case, who was rushed into hospital with his leg, actually went home to feed his chickens first, before he got on a bus to go to the hospital, in order to attend the appointment that I had arranged for him at the Vascular Studies Clinic, later that afternoon.

Now that I think about it, this chap's daughter may well have actually said, 'That GP was a rum 'un. He turned round to mi dad and said, "You look starved. Put that barm cake down, 'cos I'm rushing you to hospital."'

Ivan

By the time I met Ivan, he was disabled and housebound. He had been born with achondroplasia, the commonest genetic cause of very short stature. Despite the limitations of his condition, he had made the best of things and forged a career in entertainment, being part of a musical comedy duo. He had appeared on variety shows throughout the UK, often touring with famous musicians and comedians. He had also worked in Las Vegas for several years and still had the photographs of leisure time spent relaxing by swimming pools, with members of the Rat Pack and various showgirls. He had later moved back to his home town, as his health deteriorated, to be near his family. During my home visits, he was happy to show me photographs of his better times, mostly in the 1960s, and I was happy to look at them and to hear his stories.

Of more pressing urgency was his search for more suitable adapted accommodation. He had faced several barriers in gaining support from the local council's housing department, chiefly that they had awarded him zero points on their illness and disability scorecard. It appeared that he needed fifteen points to be allowed a move to a suitably adapted flat. He was baffled and had asked me for help. One problem with this was that the council had never given GPs information on their scoring system, so it was hard to help needy patients to increase their score and chances of moving. Ivan later told me that he'd rung the appropriate office in the council and had spoken to the lady who'd initially rejected his rehousing application.

He said, 'I asked her why she had not given me any points for my two conditions. She said that they weren't on her list.

I asked if she knew what they meant and she didn't, as she had no medical qualifications. I told her what the back problem meant, but she still said that wasn't enough. I then asked her about my achondroplasia.'

'She said, "What's that?"

'I said, "I'm a dwarf."

'She said, "What's a dwarf?"

'I said, "Have you ever watched *Snow White and the Seven Dwarves*?"

'She said, "Yes."

'I said, "I'm one of those. I'll send you a photograph."

'And I did. A signed one. I got a letter saying I now had sixteen points and I'm moving next month, when they finish my new kitchen off. I rang her yesterday and she's put my photo on the wall near her desk. She loves me now and can't do enough to help.'

I was reminded of Ivan when I found one of his photographs in a pile of papers I was sorting out last week. It was a photograph of all the members of a touring variety show, together with a mayor and lady mayoress, all of them overlooking a fine seaside promenade. On the photo were numerous musicians and comedians, famous from the sixties onwards. In the centre of the picture, at the very front, was Ivan, smiling broadly. He had done well, at a time when I suspect things were even harder for people who looked different or had any disabilities.

Albert

Albert limped into my consulting room. He was in his mid-sixties, had a full beard and a fuller smile. He had no walking stick or frame.

I broke the ice: 'What's up with your leg?'

Albert replied, smile growing wider, 'I don't know; I've not seen it for years. It's in a jar at Manchester Royal.'

He sat down and pulled up his right trouser leg. I could now clearly see his tin leg. I apologised for my tactless question, but he would not accept it.

'It's just my little joke, Doc, don't worry.'

Albert had extensive and serious arterial disease throughout his body, and had had this for years. His leg had required a below-knee amputation because of this disease while he was only in his forties. He also had significant heart disease, having had several heart attacks and ongoing angina. He continued to smoke, despite this exacerbating his inbuilt genetic tendency to severe arterial problems. Like many tobacco addicts, he claimed that smoking was his only pleasure and, fatalistically (and incorrectly), 'There's no point in stopping 'cos the damage is already done.'

By the time he first started consulting me, we fortunately had some stronger medications available to try to help him, so there was some hope. Statins had not been out long but had been shown to be far more effective than the previous cholesterol-lowering drugs available. Albert continued to see a number of different specialists and all of these were for problems related to his under-lying arterial problems.

Over time, his walking became worse and he had trouble with his stump and prosthesis. He was using two elbow crutches within a few years, but still continued to drive his suitably adapted car and to see me in the surgery. He was always such a cheerful man, even as he deteriorated generally. His angina and subsequent heart failure became worse, and it appeared that the statins had arrived a bit too late to have any massive impact on his arteries, although the smoking obviously did not help.

During one Friday evening surgery, I was summoned from my room to the rainy street outside. Albert's car had hit a lamp post, which was now leaning over slightly. The car engine was still running and revving quite loudly. By the car stood a few staff from the next-door chemist and one of our receptionists. We opened the car door. Albert was slumped to the side and leaning forward. He was unresponsive. I turned the car engine off and then hauled him from the car onto the wet pavement. I asked the receptionist to call a 999 ambulance. One of the practice nurses had joined me by then and we performed CPR for five minutes before the rain started to fall more heavily. I made the decision to take him into the surgery, five yards away. I did not like the idea of this lovely man ending his time on Earth on the pavement, watched by the customers in the chemist and also passengers gawping at him from the buses stopping at the nearby traffic lights.

We carried him into my room; me holding his body while the nurse supported his legs, flesh and tin. We put him onto the examination couch and resumed our CPR attempts, this time with the benefit of oxygen. We did not yet have a defibrillator at that time. The ambulance crew arrived soon after and we used their portable ECG to assess Albert's status. There was no fibrillation or heartbeat of any kind. We admitted defeat and covered him up. The police were informed and the ambulance crew waited for them to arrive so they could remove the body.

I still had most of my evening surgery to complete, although I was well over an hour late. There were twelve patients already sitting in the waiting room and a few more still to arrive. I would need to speak to the police when they arrived, hopefully soon. We decided to ask any patients if they could come in on the Monday instead and I would see them then, unless it was absolutely urgent for that evening. Thankfully, everybody bar one patient agreed to come back. Most of them had seen some of the comings and goings on the pavement and in my room so realised it was quite serious. The police arrived and I spoke to them before Albert's body was removed by the ambulance crew. It was an unexpected death but there were no suspicious circumstances. Albert had apparently called at the chemist for his prescription, then got in his car and driven slowly just a few yards into the lamp post.

The 'emergency' patient waited in the waiting room until the police and ambulance crew, with poor Albert, left around 8 p.m. I saw this solitary patient in a colleague's room, adjacent to mine, because of all the debris and detritus still left in mine. His emergency was very mild penile thrush and could not wait until the Monday, apparently. Go figure, as Americans say.

No Girls Allowed

One of the features of General Practice in the 1990s and early 2000s was the frequent changes to the NHS organisational structures, nationally and locally. Associated with this were frequent new management initiatives for primary care, usually incorporating the latest ideas from America about improving efficiency and teamwork. In order to accommodate these ideas, we were encouraged to take part in many practice awaydays, often including an overnight stay at a nice hotel. The attendees included the GPs, nurses, administration and reception teams. We were even given grants towards the costs of these training and brainstorming courses, run by enthusiastic gurus with their bright ideas and striped shirts. We tried to forget our cynicism a bit and tried to become enthused, and we certainly enjoyed the opportunity to think, in a protected space with time away from real work. We certainly also enjoyed the nice food and hotels.

I remember one such meeting at a nice hotel in Cheshire. We had just finished our morning session and were walking over towards the landing area where we expected to have our buffet lunch. There were already some people there, picking at the food.

Picking at our food.

They were all young women and had their backs to us. The other thing of note was that they were really quite vociferous and were also swearing noisily. A lot.

A few of the girls turned round as we approached. They looked quite glamorous and also quite familiar.

Just then, an older man appeared through the ballroom doorway and shouted, 'You're in here, girls! That's somebody else's.'

The girls walked off through the doorway, without looking back. They were the pop group Girls Aloud. Appropriately named and quite famous, as they were the winners of a recent BBC TV series; but not as famous then as they were to become over the next decade.

It was a brief encounter of sorts but a funny one for us at the time – 'Girls Aloud nicked our buffet.'

I remembered this incident when I heard the sad news about the death of Sarah Harding, aged only thirty-nine, in 2021.

'Your Three O'Clock'

'Dr S, your three o'clock appointment, Angela, is on the phone. Can you speak to her now, as she can't come in?' asked Kelly, one of the receptionists.

'Err, yeah, I suppose so,' I said, trying to access Angela's computer records before the call was put through. 'Why can't she come in?'

'She can tell you herself. I'll put her through.' Click.

'Hello, is that Dr S?' said Angela.

'Yes. Are you OK?' I replied.

'I'm OK, ta,' she replied through a lot of background noise.

'I just wondered, as you normally come into the surgery,' I said questioningly.

'I'm in hospital and they won't let me out yet.'

'Oh dear, sorry to hear that. What's up?' I asked.

'I took a paracetamol overdose last night and I'm on a drip to help.'

'Gosh, that doesn't sound good. Is it Parvolex* in the drip?' I asked.

'Yes, something like that.'

'And how are you feeling now?' I asked.

'I'm a bit tired 'cos you can't get any peace on these wards at night. You know what it's like.'

I did.

'How do you feel about the overdose now?' I asked.

'Oh, I'd just had a fallin' out and drunk too much. Not like last time,' she replied.

---

* This was the brand name of a drug used to try to prevent liver damage following a paracetamol overdose.

'OK, and have they arranged for you to see any of the psychiatric team yet?' I asked.

'Yeah, but that's not what I've rung for.'

'OK. How can I help you then?' I asked, slightly confused.

'I just wondered what my cholesterol was?'

'Sorry?'

'I had my bloods done yesterday morning at the surgery,' she said.

'Oh, right. I see.'

I saw. The results were fine. She did not need to take a statin, as had been considered at her last surgery appointment with a colleague. I told her the results and reassured her.

'You can't too careful.'

Said the lady who had ostensibly just tried to kill herself, about considering medication to give her some possible potential long-term future health protection.

It was hard to see much logic in her impulsive behaviour and concerns over the previous twenty-four hours, but perhaps some reassurance that she was not currently planning on another immediate suicide attempt. Unless she had a drink and fell out again, of course.

Reflections on Practice

You might think that the hardest part of being a doctor, generally, and a GP, specifically, when confronted with a patient is making a diagnosis. This is not the case. It is not that the diagnosis is always easy: it isn't. It is just that the diagnosis is not always important or essential, at least at the first consultation. The main issue is often managing uncertainty, and working out a suitable plan with the patient's consent and agreement.

Many diagnoses become more obvious with time or with the arrival of the results from blood tests and other investigations. Trainee GPs often struggle with this uncertainty, as they are used to the ready and instant availability of blood tests and scan results when they worked in hospitals. Their other distraction and concern is often, what I call, FOMAS (fear of missing a syndrome). This occurs when a patient has a few different symptoms or signs and the trainee has a niggling feeling that there may be one single diagnosis that explains all of these. This feeling is a bit of a hangover from hospital training posts when there is always another clever* doctor hanging over their shoulder, waiting to show their intellectual and medical superiority with a sudden cry of, 'It's obviously Volksberg-Engelheim† syndrome.'

As stated, sometimes a time delay can help. I remember my trainer telling me that the best way to diagnose Parkinson's disease or hypothyroid disease‡ in patients was to go on holiday

---

* Smart-arse.
† Not a real syndrome or disease, I don't think. Unless I'm missing something …
‡ Commonly known as 'underactive' thyroid.

and let your colleague make the diagnosis. There is certainly some truth in this, as often the signs and symptoms of these, and many other, conditions can develop so slowly and gradually that you may miss them if you see the patient too frequently.

Another issue is dealing with patient expectations, starting with the expectation of never becoming ill and the rightful anger that many people feel at developing disease. I believe that people often accepted illness as their lot more often in the past than now. Times were often hard. Many of our parents or grandparents still remember a time before antibiotics and before the development of many of the vaccinations we have now against communicable disease. People suffered from diseases such as polio, diphtheria and also TB. There were no effective treatments for these diseases other than isolating people in remote hospitals and hoping they got better before passing their infections on any further.

Thankfully, in many ways, we now expect good health as our right, and illness can be a massive shock in this context, especially for younger people, of course. Supporting patients through the shock and acceptance of their symptoms and conditions is a big part of the GP's work.

The hardest struggle of all can be for those who are carers for family members with disease and disability. They often have little hope of things getting any easier, and can be overwhelmed and exhausted by their lives, with little prospect of much time off and insufficient outside support. Seeing carers in their roles makes many of doctors' complaints of long hours and overwork seem relatively trivial. I often felt humbled in the presence of many of the carers I met. At least I could go home and relax later.

Carry On, Doctor

Our practice did not usually have much need to employ locum doctors, as there were six GP partners who could generally cover for each other's holidays or sick leave. The exception tended to be when partners took maternity leave and we employed long-term locums at these times. One of these was Dr Jessop, who was a good and conscientious doctor. He was, however, young, shy and easily embarrassed.

Over coffee one morning, he blushed while he told me about an awkward moment during one of his consultations in his earlier morning surgery. An elderly lady, Jean, was telling him about her breathlessness and he was trying to clarify when she was affected by this.

'What are you like when you're walking indoors?' he asked.

'I'm OK, apart from when I go up the stairs.'

'What are you like in bed?' he continued.

'Well, I've never had any complaints,' replied Jean.

Cue Dr Jessop's blushing, which continued for the rest of the morning, especially as I continually asked him to recount his story to the other GPs as they came in for coffee.

A few days later, he told me of another consultation. This one was with a young woman who requested medication for acne, but wondered if she could be prescribed a particular brand of contraceptive pill that she had read about as being effective for both contraception and skin problems.

'Are you sexually active?' Dr Jessop asked her.

'Err, not really. I usually just lie there and he does most of the work.' Honest, at least, if not especially romantic.

Despite his easy discomfort, Dr Jessop continued as a maternity-cover locum for a few more months before he started in a permanent GP post somewhere in Cheshire. I hope and expect that his shyness has eased a bit, otherwise he faces a lifetime of embarrassment in his chosen career path.

Gifts

Stories abound of grateful patients leaving their GPs large gifts in their wills. At least they do among older or retired GPs, who tell these tales with a wistful, maybe jealous, look in their embittered eyes. There would obviously be moral and ethical worries about any large gifts, and anything above £100 value now needs to be registered by GPs in England. None of the kind gifts I received over the years approached this figure. The idea of such generous gifts to GPs took a more sinister turn in the 1990s with the unfolding story of Dr Shipman, who was caught and investigated for his mass murders because he attempted to forge a will. Doctor Shipman was a GP thought to have murdered an estimated 250 victims. We worked in his shadow to some extent, as his practice was only four miles away from ours and some of his victims were relatives of my patients. Other patients often had a fairly black sense of humour and frequently referred to 'that Shipman and his evil deeds' in a lighter fashion than was really appropriate:

'Are you sure it's just a flu jab in that syringe, Doc? Only I don't have a lot of money,' was heard on more than one occasion during the flu-jab season.

I was visiting another patient, Ida, at her nice home a few miles from the surgery.

'That's a nice car you've got there,' she said, peering at it through her net curtains.

'Thank you; I like it, anyway,' I said. It was a decent three-year-old, four-wheel-drive car.

'Would you like a better one sometime?' she asked, instantly deflating my preening.

'One day, maybe, when this one's paid off,' I muttered.

'I could always leave you a posh one in my will,' she teased.

'No, thanks, I don't think that's a good idea,' I replied.

'I suppose not. They'd be digging me up again when they found out. I'm sure you're right,' she said with a smile. Several district nurses later told me that she had a similar conversation with them.

Two of my GP friends who worked in a nearby village were once invited to the reading of a will of one of their deceased patients. They sat, with his family and several of his old friends, in a local solicitor's office. One by one, the details of property, land, cash and gifts were read out and gratefully received. The last two gifts were for the expectant medics, who were sat quietly at the back of the office. Dr Austin was left a small framed photograph of the village. Dr Astley was left a half-bottle of whisky. To be precise, this was half of a full bottle of whisky, rather than a new half-bottle. Neither of them were especially thrilled but were allegedly relieved that they had avoided the wrath of the family or friends from being left anything of excess value. That was their story, anyway.

Many patients did actually give me a bottle of wine or even whisky at Christmas, and these were always full. The patients who gave these kind gifts tended to be naturally generous souls rather than regular attenders or receivers of much medical care.

Gone Fishing

Christopher, a man in his mid-forties, was referred to me by one of the practice nurses following his routine blood tests. His tests revealed an alarmingly high, fasting total cholesterol reading of 12 mmol/L.* A blood cholesterol reading comprises a list of the different type of fats, known as lipids. These include different types of cholesterol and also triglycerides. The ratio of these different components can help with prediction of future heart disease risk and helps to guide the consideration of whether or not to consider prescribing a statin for an individual. Statins are brilliant drugs for reducing unsafe cholesterol levels and, consequently, heart disease in the vulnerable. They are prescribed in high numbers in the UK and have gained some bad publicity based on reported side effects. More recent trials have shown much lower side effects and drug withdrawals than those originally reported in the nineties and noughties.

I cannot remember the full breakdown on this chap's lipid readings, but the headline total cholesterol figure of 12 was shockingly high on its own, compared to a UK average of 5.7. Christopher already seemed to have some awareness of the significance of his blood test and had additionally read up a little bit about it before his appointment. I remember trying to push him towards a statin early on in the consultation rather than establishing his thoughts and expectations first, as is best practice.

'I don't want one of those bloody drugs,' said Christopher. 'I'll put myself on a diet and it'll come down.'

---

* A normal total cholesterol would be 5mmol/L or lower; even lower still if the person is already known to be at high risk of cardiovascular disease.

I pursed my lips and breathed out, in the manner of a mechanic or a plumber before breaking bad news. 'It's not going to come down far enough. The most you can manage with even a really good diet is about twenty per cent reduction and you need at least fifty.'

'I'll do it. Let me try a diet for three months and then do the tests again,' he said.

I felt it unlikely but agreed. I didn't have much choice to be fair, as his mind was made up. He was certainly well motivated, but did not want to discuss the specifics of his current or planned diet.

'I'll show you,' he said, smiling at me as he left the room.

I smiled back and thought, *we'll see*, to myself, smugly.

Six point five. That was Christopher's repeat fasting total cholesterol a little over three months later. I was stunned but, honestly, really pleased for him.

'Well, Doc, how's about that, then?' he asked on the way into my room, speaking in the manner of a now discredited, criminal, deceased former DJ and television personality.

'Absolutely brilliant. How on earth did you manage that?' I asked.

'I knew I would do it. You didn't believe me, did you?' It was his turn to bask in smugness, this time well-earned.

I had to admit my doubts and surprise, and asked him again what he had done.

'Well, you know I came into a bit of money a few years ago? No? Well, I did. So I packed up work and basically spend just about every day fishing. I love it.'

'That's good, but what's that got to do with your cholesterol?' I asked.

He smiled and went on, reeling me in. 'Well, I don't like cooking, so I have a chippy dinner and a chippy tea, and then a chippy supper on the way home from the pub.'

After a few moments to take all that in, I said, 'Gosh. So have you given up the chippy and the beer now?'

'No, but I stopped having supper from the chippy. I still have my dinner and tea there, but I also now have more fish than pies.'

I still doubted that just dropping one out of three chip-shop meals could make such a massive impact on his cholesterol, but the proof of the (beef) pudding appeared to be in its non-eating. I congratulated him again and we agreed to retest his lipids in a further three months. The cholesterol rose a little, but he brought it down again for the following time.

I have not seen him for a while, so am not sure what his current cholesterol and chip-shop status is. I did marvel at his apparent lack of ambition with his financial windfall, but each to his own, and I hope he stays well enough to enjoy his prolonged leisure time.

My own diet was generally, in those days, a bit better than Christopher's; certainly at lunchtime, anyway. I usually left the surgery for a short walk around the town, to buy a sandwich and also clear my head a little before the afternoon or evening surgeries. One of the practice cleaners, Clare, told me that she had seen me walking around with my lunch and asked me why I never called into the café in the local indoor market. She worked there as well as at our surgery.

I replied – 'I never thought about it, really.'

Clare – 'Well you should. It's good grub.'

Me – 'I try to avoid having a big lunch, as I might feel too sleepy in the afternoon. I also want to eat more healthy stuff than fry-ups, as well.'

Clare – 'We do healthy food as well.'

Me – 'Oh, yes. Like what?'

Clare – 'We do salads.'

Me – 'Oh, that sounds better. What kind of salads do you do?'

Clare – 'We do a pie salad. Oh, and a pasty salad.'

Me, laughing – 'That doesn't sound very healthy.'

Clare, now smiling – 'Well, it's a nice pie and a nice salad, anyway.'

I thanked her and said that I might try it one day, but – perhaps, sadly – I never did.

Gratitude?

Many patients are extremely appreciative and grateful for the efforts that the NHS and its staff make on their behalf: thanks also to the development of new drugs and technologies that have made previously terminal illnesses now curable. Perhaps, sometimes, we are all guilty of taking such things for granted. I certainly remember a few patients who seemed a bit less grateful than you might expect.

One of these was Wilf, who had developed renal (kidney) failure during his fifties and sixties. His renal function became so seriously impaired that he required dialysis in hospital. This life-saving and life-prolonging treatment was an immense triumph of technology and effort but, to be fair, is a nuisance for patients, who soon got bored of spending the best part of three days a week connected to a dialysis machine. It also involved lots of other appointments with specialists and nurses and dieticians and phlebotomists, and also a very restricted diet. Wilf was generally a miserable person before his illness, but became significantly more miserable during his treatment, especially after he started dialysis. I had some sympathy for him. Living with such a severe condition and also the impact of the treatment itself must be really difficult and exhausting. Even travelling to the regional renal unit itself was a trial for him too as, at that time, the local hospital did not have a dialysis unit and home units were only just being considered. He felt angry at having renal disease and felt trapped by his time pinned to the machine.

Wilf's luck picked up; he was put forward for a transplant and waited only a short time for a suitable kidney to become available and implanted. He still required regular anti-rejection medications and close follow-up at the renal unit, but would not require to be plugged in for three days a week. I saw his name on my appointment list a few months after his successful transplant and I looked forward to seeing him. I called him into my room and we both sat down.

I beamed a smile at him and said, 'How are you doing?'

'OK,' he muttered grudgingly. 'I suppose.'

'Really? I thought you'd be feeling much better now,' I said, trying to initiate some enthusiasm.

'I feel completely abandoned, to be honest.'

'What do you mean? Has something gone wrong?' I asked, now wondering if I had missed some update from the hospital.

'They've just abandoned me, completely.'

'What do you mean?' I asked.

'Well, they don't want to see me now.'

'Isn't that a good thing? You used to get fed up going there so much of the time,' I suggested.

'No. They just don't care anymore. I'm on the scrapheap,' he said and sighed.

'You've got the amazing gift of a new kidney from some poor bugger who has died and you'd rather go back to dialysis?' I said disbelievingly.

'It would be better than being ignored,' he said.

Unbelievable. He remained ungrateful about his new kidney whenever I saw him over the next few years.

Piotr was an NHS radiographer who had originally arrived in the UK from Poland some ten years ago. He had married a British-born midwife and had two small children. He presented at the surgery with a suspicious hard lump in the right axilla (armpit) and was referred on a two-week urgent basis for investigation. Shortly after referral, he developed another lump.

Biopsies confirmed a type of lymphoma and Piotr was referred on to a regional oncology (cancer) unit for further treatment. For a while, the oncologists struggled with a precise diagnosis and appropriate treatment regime, and Piotr became seriously ill until the disease eventually responded well to a newer chemo-therapy treatment course. During that time he had continued to develop further lumps, which raised everybody's anxiety levels even more. His wife had kept us up to date about all this when she came to the surgery a few times for her or her children's appointments. It had obviously been a dreadful and immensely worrying time for Piotr and his family.

I had recently seen a clinic letter from his oncologist, thank-fully confirming that Piotr was now effectively disease-free and was being returned to routine follow-up only. Piotr came to see me about another matter.

As he walked in, I congratulated him on his progress and he smiled back broadly and said, 'I know. It's brilliant. I've even got most of my hair back now. More than you've got, anyway.'

It was hard to begrudge him a mild mickey-take at my expense, especially as he was correct. The consultation then continued on another matter and towards the end I issued him with a prescription for medication he'd requested. He stood up to leave. I asked him when he was restarting work.

He replied, 'I'm not sure yet. I might not go back to the hospital,' and then, 'I'm suing the NHS.'

'What? Why?' I replied, my smile now gone.

'Because we were told I was going to die and I didn't, of course.'

'Well, surely that's good news?' I asked, still bewildered.

'Yes, but not really. When they told us I was likely to die, we cashed in my pension.'

'Well, can't you pay that money back in and start again?' I asked.

'No, we spent it on a new kitchen and doing up the house. My family have got no savings left.'

'OK. Sorry to hear that, but they've got you; your wife's got a husband and your kids have still got a dad. Isn't that better? You're still young,' I tried.

He was irritated with me now and said, 'I'm not suing them because they cured me. I'm suing them because they said they couldn't. Anyway, it's with my lawyers now and I don't want to talk about it. Thanks for the prescription.' He left.

Being empathic to patients' situations is an essential part of being a GP. It does not mean that you have to agree with them or their outlook, but it should allow you to try to understand the world through their eyes and current perspective. Try as I might, I could not put myself in a position where I would be angry enough with the NHS (or other healthcare provider) that I would want to sue them for saving my life, especially if my wife and I worked for them. Maybe my empathy muscles have worn out.

Dan

One of the practice regulars was Dan. He was an alcoholic and often attended surgery requesting diazepam or other tranquillisers, especially when he had run out of money for booze. Drugs like these seemed to be prescribed quite often by GPs in the 1970s and early 1980s, but from then on we tried to resist prescribing them and spent a lot of time and effort trying to help patients reduce and stop them. This was, understandably, hard work, as these drugs are very addictive. Dan was often very friendly and quite likeable, unless he attended while steaming drunk. On one of the latter occasions, he turned up at the reception on a Friday evening, demanding to be seen by the duty doctor. That was me. The reception staff dealt with him politely, saying that the duty doctor was seeing emergency problems only and that he should attend for his routine booked appointment the following week. He tried again, telling them that he felt really ill and was in a bad way, and it was an emergency. Once again he was gently rebuffed and he walked away from the reception desk and sat down in the front row of the waiting-room chairs.

One of the receptionists popped out of the reception area to get me to sign a bundle of prescriptions. Dan seized his opportunity. He jumped up and scuttled through the door into reception before it closed and locked again. He grabbed a small, round, black container from the reception desk and announced, 'I'm gonna take the fuckin' lot of these if you don't get me an appointment with the doc!'

The nearest receptionist, Sue, looked at him, bemused, and said, 'You'll be lucky. They're urine testing strips.'

Dan looked back at the bottle, laughed and tried pleading again instead of threatening. It was no good. Sue was still laughing and he had lost all of his impetus.

Dan walked away saying, 'Oh, I'm off.'

A few years later, Dan came to see me at a booked appointment. He strode in confidently, looking quite smart.

'Good morning,' I said. 'How're you?'

'I'm good. I've retired today.'

I nearly choked on the coffee I had just slurped. I coughed and then sniggered out loud.

'What're you laughing at? I have retired. Today,' he said.

'Retired from what?' I asked. 'You haven't worked for thirty years!'

'Ah, don't be like that, Doc,' he said.

'Well, are you gonna stop boozing now? Is that it? Career over?'

'No, don't be daft, of course not,' he said and chuckled. 'I just get me pension now so won't need any more sick notes. I'm sixty-five.'

I wished him a happy birthday, of course. I can't remember what he had booked his appointment for that day, but I do remember him telling me that he was heading off to meet his mates in the pub to celebrate his birthday and new status.

Sports Medic

In 1997, all GPs within thirty miles of Manchester were sent a letter asking if they would like to be involved in providing medical support at the Commonwealth Games, coming to the city in 2002. I was keen and replied suitably, awaiting my next instructions. In 2000, I received a follow-up letter asking if I was still interested. I had forgotten about the first letter but my interest was reignited and I replied suitably again.

In 2001, we received our first instructions to attend a training session near the nearly completed City of Manchester Stadium, now known as the Etihad Stadium. The training was focused on introducing us to the principles of sports medicine, particularly on authorised versus non-authorised medications for athletes. We were given talks by sports doctors, pharmacists and also athletes themselves. Many of the speakers and staff were Australians who had been, wisely, brought in from the team that ran the brilliant Sydney Olympics in 2000. It was clear that the Aussies had a vastly superior and more professional administrative sports set-up than the UK at that time.

Manchester had bid to be the host city for the Olympics twice and failed twice. The Commonwealth Games were originally seen as a consolation prize, but were fully embraced by the city and the volunteer programme was overwhelmed with applicants.

I was to be a part of the general medical team based in the Athlete's Village at Owen's Park, responsible for providing medical backup for the smaller teams who did not have their own medics and physiotherapists, as well as medical support at each of the venues. We were also responsible for providing general support for the technical staff and the attendant VIPs and VVIPs* (their official title).

The medical centre was well equipped, with an MRI scanner and a pharmacy and numerous clinic and physiotherapy suites. There were some A&E consultants on the rota but most of the medics were GPs. There was also dental and ophthalmology teams present who were incredibly busy throughout – it being a little-known responsibility of the organisers to provide good dental and eye care for all members of the attending teams. Many of the athletes and coaches from smaller and poorer countries had a lot of non-urgent dental work during their stay and many left with their maximum allowance of two new pairs of glasses.

The Village and medical centre were already active a few weeks before the Games themselves and became busier as the opening ceremony approached. We ate our meals in the main food tent, alongside the athletes, which added to the excitement and feeling of belonging.

In the clinic sessions, we typically saw routine things such as tonsillitis, contraception requests, rashes and tummy upsets. The athletes were obviously more driven than my usual patients and very focused, especially on being fit for their competition days.

I saw a girl who had a painful heel. I listened to her explanation of symptoms and likely causes, then examined her, and we then talked about a treatment plan. She was a long jumper, and had bruised her heel on an awkward landing.

I asked her, 'Do you want a steroid injection?'†

---

* Very, Very Important Person/People.
† Localised injections of corticosteroids are allowed for athletes and are not considered to be a form of doping. These are usually a combination of a local anaesthetic and long-acting steroid, which reduces pain and inflammation. Older patients often tend to refer to them as 'cortisone' injections. The more worrying and banned types of steroids are anabolic steroids which, broadly, promote the development of muscles and strength.

'No, it's OK. I'll just go for that physio and take those tablets that you're prescribing [ibuprofen],' she replied politely.

'Do you still have any competitive sessions left?' I asked, wondering why she appeared to be in less of a rush than most of the previous patients I had seen that morning.

'No, it's fine. I've finished, thank you. I'll go and get these now.' She left, waving at me with the script.

When I arrived home later that night after my shift, I sat and watched some of the Games highlights, including the ladies' long jump competition. The girl I had seen that morning had won a medal. She hadn't mentioned it during the consultation. She had also limped away from the long jump pit after her last jump, with her sore heel already evident.

Another clinic patient was a young, chatty Anglo-Pakistani weightlifter from the midlands. He was representing Pakistan rather than England, in order to make his dad proud. He had developed acute pain in his shoulder, which was affecting his ability to lift his normal competition weight. He was due to compete later that day and was keen for me to give him a steroid injection, which I did. Later that night, I was pleased to see him on TV, winning a medal.

I was also scheduled to do a few clinics at both the technical support accommodation and later, on the following day, at the Midland Hotel. Both of these clinics required me to get a bus into Manchester City Centre carrying a large cooler bag containing commonly needed drugs, as well as some medical equipment and blood-collecting gear. I was then set up, firstly in a small clinic room at the Manchester Metropolitan University, where I conducted an international GP surgery. That was interesting and involved seeing an older group of patients than the athletes, many of whom who were suffering from chronic conditions more akin to those I was more familiar with seeing at my normal surgery.

One Australian chap I saw had developed an acute liver problem; without access to his medical records, it was hard to verify his previous declared history. I suspected that he was a chronic heavy drinker who had challenged his liver a bit more than usual during his trip to Manchester. This seemed to be a common theme in the technical support teams. I took his bloods and arranged for an urgent ultrasound scan. I did not get to see his results as I was working outside of the clinic for the next few days.

The following day, at the Midland Hotel, I was given a patient appointment list for my clinic by a smartly dressed member of the VVIP support team. She told me to try to stay on time as these patients were not used to being kept waiting. No pressure there, then. I walked across the landing to call my first patient in and was slightly starstruck on seeing a few British former Olympic medallists stood around talking to each other, and also some familiar TV presenters. They looked right through me and I looked past them to my first patient, who I called and then accompanied back to the room. He and the other patients I saw that morning were either high-ranking politicians or very high-ranking sports officials from Commonwealth countries, of course. Once again, this was very different to my normal workplace, but people are people in the end, even if they are smartly dressed, and don't like waiting.

I noticed that one of my patients that day was from Botswana. A member of the support team had gone to fetch him as he was not in the waiting area. He knocked and came in. I greeted him in Setswana. He stood open-mouthed for a few moments before stuttering his reply, and then smiled broadly and switched into English, thankfully.

'I was not expecting that. You have surprised me! Have you been to my country?'

I told him that I had, when I was a medical student, and had worked in a hospital there for a few months. He seemed pleased, but we then moved on quickly to his health concerns, as you would expect. He kindly suggested that I should contact him if I ever went back to Botswana and gave me a card with his details on.

Towards the end of the Games a raffle was held in the medical centre; the prize was the opportunity to attend the closing ceremony in the main stadium. I was one of the randomly chosen few who were bussed to the stadium on the last night. It was tremendously exciting and good fun, despite the heavy rain. We walked out onto the pitch after the massed Mini Minors during the parades. We also got to stay on the pitch for the trippy dance music and firework show at the very end.

I had really enjoyed my time volunteering at the Games and the small part I got to play in things. It was good to see a completely different set of patients than usual.

It would be more difficult to get involved in the same way nowadays, as I understand that sports medicine diplomas or other extra qualifications are now required for this sort of work.

I had also been impressed by the complex planning and organisational skills that had gone into the event. An (unexpected) volunteer medal arrived in the post about six months later.

Look – It's Gone!

I'm sure that most doctors and nurses can identify with patients turning up after the event, so to speak. Many patients turn up for appointments and describe long-gone rashes and symptoms. Often this is inevitable, as these things can happen in the night or at weekends or there can be problems getting an appointment when you want one. Sometimes there is still a point in still sharing information on such rashes or symptoms because of ongoing related disease, but very often there isn't. Many are the times that appointments are booked for rashes or spots that disappeared days or even weeks ago.

'What do you think it was?' asked the patient.

'I'm not sure. Did you take a picture?'

'No.'

'Well, as it has now gone it is very unlikely to have been anything serious,' I tried to reassure him.

'How can you be sure?' he said, still not completely reassured.

'Well, it can't be the melanoma that you're worried about as it has gone.'

He tried again. 'What do I do if it comes back or I get another one?'

'I suggest you take a photo of it, ideally with a tape measure or coin next to it so we can judge the size, and book a routine review appointment if it persists and you are worried about it.'

Quite a palaver for a spot, which had already gone before he'd even booked his appointment.

On another occasion, I came back to work after being off on sick leave for a month. One of our regulars, Mary, had booked in to see me. She was a remarkably active lady in her mid-nineties who regularly attended the surgery for appointments; she still took frequent cruise ship holidays in the Caribbean and Far East, and later entertained GPs and nurses with tales from her most recent trip and plans for her next.

'My left shoulder has been really painful again and I thought you might give me a steroid injection.'

'Let me have a look at it and we'll see if that might help,' I suggested.

'It's better now,' she replied.

'That's good,' I said hopefully.

'Not really. I wanted you to see it when it was really bad,' she countered.

'Surely you're pleased that it's OK now?' I asked, hopeful again.

'No. I wish it was still bad so you could see it and inject it,' she said resentfully.

'Well, I'm pleased that it has got better. Is there anything else I can help you with while you're here?' I asked.

'No. Just that. I can't believe you were off that long. It's cost me ten pounds to get a taxi here and now it's better. Don't be going off again.'

I hoped not to be. Unless I could be off long enough for her to get better without any medical intervention, of course.

Kids, Eh?

Patients: husband and wife, Edward and Fiona. They were both also under the care of the drug team and on a methadone programme. They were in their mid-forties but looked much older. Fiona, in particular, also had some additional chronic physical and mental health problems. They had arrived thirty minutes late for their appointments but persuaded our receptionists that they were still worthy of being squeezed into my, now even more delayed, surgery.

Edward – 'Sorry, we're late. We had to wait for a taxi. Our Tom's [their son] had his car taken off him by the cops.'

Fiona – 'It's ridiculous.'

Me – 'Why have they done that?'

Edward – ''Cos it's stolen.'

Fiona – 'It's not fair.'

Edward – 'I mean, it's only a teenage thing.'

Me – 'What is?'

Edward – 'Nickin' a car. I mean, we've all done it.'

Me – 'I haven't.'

Edward – 'Course you have. Just kids being kids.'

Me – 'Not me.'

Edward – 'It's nothing.'

Fiona – 'They're just victimising him 'cos they know us.'

Me – 'Did he actually steal the car?'

Edward – 'Yeah, but he's looked after it better than they did.'

Fiona – 'They don't deserve a nice car, people like that.'

Me – 'People like what?'

Edward – 'People with money. It all comes a bit easy for 'em and they don't appreciate things like we do.'

Me – 'Maybe it's not easy for them if they've had to work hard to save up or borrow the money!'

Fiona – 'You would be on their side.'

Me – 'I'm happy to help you, but I don't have to agree with everything you say. Shall we get on?'

Edward – 'How do you get one of those Motability* cars?'

Me – 'Apart from nicking one?'

Edward, laughing now – 'I suppose there is that, but how do you get a proper one?'

Me – 'Well, you start off by having a disability.'

Fiona – 'We have. We've got addiction.'

Me – 'That doesn't count.'

Fiona – 'And bad knees.'

Me – 'They're not bad enough.'

Edward, shaking his head and looking serious – 'So the only way for us to get a car really is to nick one.'

Me – 'Or get a job and buy one.'

Edward – 'Be serious.'

I thought I was. Fortunately, we then moved on to a different, slightly more medical tack from then on, for that afternoon at least.

---

* The Motability scheme is an affordable way for disabled people to lease a new car by exchanging their mobility allowance for it. It is generally regarded as a very good deal, as it covers all motoring costs except fuel. In some very disadvantaged areas, many of the newer cars you see are very likely to be Motability cars.

Misunderstood

Brian was an occasional attendee. He was a semi-retired architect and a bit of a raconteur. After dealing with his or his in-laws' medical problems, he would chat with me about the latest guitars he had bought: mostly antique, high-end models. I, too, have a keen interest in music and had a few nice guitars of my own, although none with the provenance and price tags of his. On another occasion, while we were waiting for the practice secretary to pop down with paperwork for a hospital referral, he told me that he was just back from a working trip to the Far East. He was involved in a few building projects over there and had also taken the opportunity to have some rest and relaxation at a variety of smart beach resorts. He then casually let slip that he had bumped into, and spoken to, Pol Pot, near one of the pools in a swish resort.

I was shocked and said: 'What? The Pol Pot? From Cambodia?'

Brian smiled. 'Yeah. He's a really nice guy.'

'But he's a genocidal dictator! I thought he was dead.'

'He's very much alive, and that's a way over-simplistic view of things.'

'Haven't you seen *The Killing Fields*?'*

'No, but as I said, he's got a different viewpoint. I'm not saying he was perfect, but I enjoyed his company. He bought me a drink.'

---

* *The Killing Fields* is a 1984 Oscar-winning biographical film set in Cambodia. A great but disturbing film.

Well, that's all right, then. The Pol Pot regime in Cambodia was one of the most barbaric and murderous in the last century, and that was a horrific list to be on. Millions of his citizens died from murder or malnutrition.

But.

He bought Brian a drink, so can't be all bad.

Nearly Famous

General Practice is not a glamorous profession, although there is some privilege in being close to patients, especially at such key points in their lives: pregnancy; birth; illness; cure; dying; death. There is also some prestige in the local community – as long as you've not been featured in any negative articles in the local news, of course.

The title of doctor can make people alter their original view of you, especially if they find this out after meeting you, and have already formed a low opinion of you, maybe because of your accent, and they are snobs. I find it useful to remain anonymous outside work, especially on holiday, and usually avoid telling people my profession or title, although it can be a useful joker to keep in reserve. It may also accord your opinion a higher rating than it may deserve if you write a letter to the editor of a national newspaper.

Apart from that, the title is usually used by others before asking you to do something for them, staff or patients, in a similar fashion to parents using your full name before telling you off.

My partner, Michelle, and I were out for a birthday meal with her closest friend, Anthea. This was our first visit to Rosso in Manchester City Centre. Rosso being a smart Italian restaurant, inside a beautiful old building, at the top of King Street. It was part-owned by Rio Ferdinand, the former Manchester United defender. It was also quite a popular haunt for local celebrities, who had their own roped-off area within, near to, but separate from, the rest of us peasants. We spotted a few *Coronation Street* actors while we were there, as well as a well-known female TV presenter and a boy-band member, who were sat together.

We had a nice meal and later headed back towards the ornate marbled reception. I turned to pick up a free pen from a glass bowl on the entrance desk. Michelle and Anthea had meanwhile already stepped out of the front door, only to find a large group of paparazzi photographers outside, leaning over some crowd barriers with long-lensed cameras. I heard my companions shouting to the photographers, asking if they wanted to take their photographs. They were waved to one side by the photographers, irritated by the distraction. It was my turn next. I pocketed my new gold-ish pen and stepped out, slightly in front of the TV presenter and boy-band member, who were also just leaving together. The flashes started going off, blinding me to where my partner and her friend were.

Suddenly, there was a loud shout from one of the paparazzi cameramen: 'Dr S! Dr S! Are you OK?'

The flashes persisted and I spotted the chap who had shouted. His colleagues continued to take photographs, perhaps thinking they should also know me. They didn't. He, however, was one of our patients and shouted his name to me. I walked towards him and he told me quickly that he was a part-time pap, then waved me out of the way, too. I walked past the barrier and looked back to see the famous couple, who I thought were still just behind me. They had actually gone back inside the restaurant, only to emerge again when the fat fool (me) had cleared out of the way of their 'surprise' photographs.

My companions were still hooting with laughter at the thought of me being recognised and papped. We stayed outside long enough to watch the mini photo shoot and then the glamorous couple get into a parked-up Mercedes VIP minibus. This drove off, closely pursued by some of the paps, including my patient, who nearly crashed into the minibus after doing an emergency getaway in his Vauxhall Astra, camera in one hand.

It was accidental near-fame, and a brief glance into another world, before dipping back into my usual world of sickness and sick notes. Sadly, Rosso closed down recently. I still have the pen. It still works.

You're Only Human, Doc

A couple in their sixties often booked consecutive appointments. Mr T (not that one) was a retired drayman and told me tales of delivering beer by horse-drawn cart when he first started in that work. Draymen were officially allowed to drink four pints a day while working, but supplemented that informally throughout the day, often having a few pints at each pub on their rounds. Unsurprisingly, he developed an alcohol-dependency problem, although this manifested itself a bit later. The beer may have been free but his marriage paid the price. He was seldom home early enough to see much of his children, at least while they were young. He had been teetotal for many years by the time I became his GP.

Mrs T was a stoical woman and had brought the children up virtually single-handedly. She had suffered from her 'nerves' as a younger woman and still had residual anxiety and depressive symptoms in her sixties. They had stayed together and were still close companions in their retirements. When they first starting seeing me, they had an allotment and I was sometimes given some of their tomatoes and leeks. They moved later into a small bungalow with a small garden, and gave the allotment up as it was a bit too far away from their new home.

Like many couples, they sat in on each other's appointments: watching and listening and chipping in with comments to help when appropriate. Usually this involved encouraging each other to tell me the full extent of their symptoms rather than downplaying the severity. Occasionally, this also involved remembering their own symptoms or medication wishes while I was conducting the consultation with their spouse. Sometimes a bit confusing, even when trying to stay on track. To try to focus their minds and remind them who was the patient, I usually asked them to change seats so that the actual current patient was sat in the nearest chair to me. Nonetheless, the potential for confusion was there.

Mrs T came to see me on a few occasions with indigestion that had not improved with over-the-counter antacids, nor with other stronger medications that I prescribed. She was resistant to any hospital referrals for investigation, particularly if this might involve 'any cameras down my throat'. She had not lost any weight or appetite and admitted that the indigestion was changing from a heartburn feeling into a cramp-like pain under her right rib edge. She was also a bit tender in that area. These symptoms were now more suggestive of gallstones, or at least some liver problem. Her blood tests for this were normal and she eventually accepted a referral for an ultrasound scan.

Around six weeks later, Mr T attended on a booked appointment. Mrs T did not have an appointment on this occasion but attended with him and sat, quietly, in the chair furthest away from mine.

'I've come for the results of my scan,' he said.

I looked at his medical records on my computer. I found an ultrasound scan report.

'Err, it's normal,'* I muttered, as I quickly scanned his records to see who had ordered this scan and what the clinical reasons were. I was a bit stumped, as I could not see any records at all relating to the scan, which was of his abdomen.

---

* It was interesting to see that Mr T had a normal-looking liver on the scan, despite his previous drinking history. This does not mean it was completely undamaged and there are more useful tests available nowadays, but he was happy to hear this and mentioned it to me at a future consultation.

'I can't seem to see who ordered this scan or why. Have you had any stomach pains?'

He looked thoughtful for a few moments, then said, 'No.'

I tried another tack. 'Do you know who ordered your scan?'

Again, 'No.'

'I'm a bit stuck,' I confessed. 'I've got no idea why you've had a scan. Do you?' This time, he shook his head from side to side while he pursed his lips.

There was an uncomfortable pause.

Then.

'My wife,' he said, and paused to clear his throat. 'My wife is waiting for a scan. We did wonder if that was anything to do with it.'

'I'm in agony, still,' said Mrs T, 'and I've not had my scan yet. Is there anything you can do to speed it up?'

My brain cogs had reluctantly started to move: rusty but now in motion.

'Right,' I started. 'I wonder if there has been some mistake and they have sent for you in error?'

'It's really hurting when I eat,' said Mrs T.

'We did wonder,' said Mr T.

'Can I ask,' I said, 'why did you go for the scan if you had nothing wrong with you?'

'We just thought it was something that I might have to do,' he replied, 'and we trust you.'

Ouch.

'Of course,' I replied. 'It's our fault. I don't know if it's mine or somebody else's yet. I'm so sorry. I'm sure we can now try to get your scan done urgently. Is that OK?' I asked Mrs T.

'You're only human, Doc,' said Mr T.

The scan, this time on the right spouse, was undertaken fairly quickly (thank you, Radiology department). It confirmed gallstones and Mrs T later saw a surgical specialist about this.

It was my fault. I had put the wrong initials on the request card and the secretary had completed the rest of the form for me, based on that error. We later reflected on this as a Significant Event at a practice meeting, and altered the way that we ordered some investigations and referrals, in order to try to minimise the opportunity for similar errors in the future.

Variety

Most GPs have other roles besides consultations and the associated paperwork and referrals. Some of these are within the practice, such as essential management and safeguarding posts and diabetic clinics, and others are within the local GP network or health authority. When I started, four of the partners in my practice also worked in hospital clinics or performing medical examinations and assessments for the Department of Social Security (DSS). Some GPs perform occupational health work for businesses. Many work for out-of-hours visit and clinic providers. Others do locum sessions at different surgeries on their days off or even when on their annual leave.

Some of my colleagues enjoy taking on the challenge of management or committee roles and will tackle a number of these. Many of the most committed give up a lot of their time, often in addition to their normal work. Some of my local colleagues have gained recognition because of this aspect of their work, eventually rising up the fountain of local, regional and national management structures. It can be tough, time-consuming, mind- and bottom-numbing work, although it can also sometimes generate its own rewards in terms of prestige and even awards, particularly, it must be said, for those also associated with political parties.

A small minority of my colleagues who take this route admit to not really enjoying consultations at all and seek out every opportunity to escape clinical work. Each to their own to some extent, and General Practice is a broad church, and its variety of roles and requirements gives it that wider appeal. Despite my cynicism, it is an absolute truth that the NHS would grind (even more) to a halt without the extraordinary efforts of doctors and others in committee and management positions.

Sadly, my eyelids tend to droop at the very mention of meeting agendas, but I had taken a strong interest in prescribing issues and was flattered into applying for, and then being elected to, a post in our local prescribing committee. We met monthly to review the newer medications and look more generally at a GP formulary, in liaison with the local hospital. It was very useful work, in theory. An example of its usefulness was the work we did in cooperation with the hospital pharmacists. For example, some drugs were much cheaper to prescribe in hospitals so were often used there, despite many of these drugs being much more expensive for primary care use. Hospital pharmacists were able to encourage the hospital doctors to initiate the use of longer-term medications that were cheaper in primary care, even if they were more expensive for the few days they were used in the hospital.

One of the peripheral roles that I did particularly enjoy was performing minor-surgery clinic sessions. I took these over when a colleague retired and continued them for the next thirty years. I really enjoyed these clinics. They were an opportunity to concentrate and focus on a single specific task with each patient. This was a vast contrast with normal surgery appointments in which you often felt a bit bombarded by the sheer number of items brought to each consultation. You had twenty to thirty minutes with each patient and clinic room staff, and were usually able to perform in a more relaxed and less rushed manner than normal, thankfully. It also allowed time to chat with the patient, clinic staff and registrars alike. I enjoyed the practical and simple skills of dissecting, excising and suturing wounds and, overall, keeping those surgical skills going. It was also a service that not every practice was able to offer to their own patients and was therefore much appreciated by ours. The clinic-staff role of setting things up and assisting was originally taken by practice nurses but became the realm and role of other trained clinic-room staff. All of them seemed to enjoy the sessions as much as I did, as they also found it a great chance to chat and laugh with patients and doctors alike. This all helped to put people at ease.

Related to this were the joint and soft-tissue injections which I, and some colleagues, did. These generally involved the use of steroids, with or without added local anaesthetic, depending on the exact injection site. The most common sites for injections tended to be shoulders, knees, elbows and heels. Patients were often very grateful for the almost instant relief offered by some of these injections and were very keen to rebook if they developed a recurrence of their condition or developed a new similar problem. As with the minor surgical clinics, I also enjoyed doing these jabs, time permitting, and in keeping these practical skills going. Both minor surgery and steroid injections required regular update courses and evidence of good practice and follow-up, but even that work was practical and more interesting than most of our other compulsory updates.

Childhood Confusion

A woman in her late twenties came to see me, accompanied by her partner, a man in his fifties. They were an unlikely couple, not just because of the age gap but because of their generational differences in clothing and speech. He was very supportive of her, in a fatherly way, I suppose. She was upset and tearful and asked if she might be referred for counselling, as this had helped her in the past. She did not feel depressed and did not want to consider any medication at that time. She told me that the cause of her stress was that she had lost a custody battle with an ex-partner and that their young daughter would now be living with this ex for most of the time, but with her still being allowed some, occasional, access.

I asked, 'Why did the courts decide that, do you think?'

'It's because I used to use a lot of drugs back in the day when I was with him,' she replied.

'Oh, I see. And is that still going on now?' I asked.

'No, I'm straight now. Colin wouldn't allow anything like that in the house,' she replied, nodding her head towards her partner, and then added, 'And I don't want to anyway.' She started sobbing, and Colin put his arm over her shoulder and pulled her towards him.

I took the opportunity to break eye contact with her and looked at her computer records. I noticed that she had two other births recorded, but only remembered her bringing one child in for emergency appointments.

'Do you have any other children?' I asked.

'No,' she said.

'Have you ever had any other children?' I asked.

'No,' she replied.

I thought about telling her why I was asking these questions but decided not to, in case she hadn't told Colin about the other children.

Colin then spoke. 'You did. You had the twins, remember?'

'Oh yeah. They were taken off me 'cos I couldn't manage them. I was too young,' she said matter-of-factly.

Very sad to think that these twins were now just a forgotten afterthought. I did not want to press her any more on this subject at the time but hoped that her counselling may give her some help. The consultation was not the right time to discuss actions, responsibility and consequences. Many of our most frequently attending patients lived in chaotic circumstances, obviously worsened if drugs were introduced into the mix. I hope that her twins had a more supportive and nourishing home environment, wherever they were, and that the younger daughter would also gain some stability in her life.

Stung

A patient, Louise, came to see me in the surgery one late autumn day. She sat down and quickly rolled up her sleeve to show me a large area of swelling and infection on her upper arm.

'I got stung a few days ago and it's getting worse,' she said.

'Gosh, that does look sore,' I responded. 'Did you see what did it?'

'Yes, it was definitely a wasp. Two days ago,' she said.

'It's a bit late in the season for stings so you are a bit unlucky,' I added.

'Well, I was away, so maybe that's it,' she said.

'Oh, where were you?' I asked, ever curious about patients' travels.

'Iceland,' she replied.

'That sounds exciting. What were you doing there?' I asked, intrigued and a bit envious.

'Buying frozen food,' she answered flatly.

'Oh, I see,' I replied, laughing. 'I thought you said you were away?'

'Yeah, I was visiting my sister in Burnley.'

Of course. Burnley frozen-food shops: the legendary haunt of late-season Lancashire wasps.

Keeping a Diary – Pre-pandemic

06:30 – Alarm goes off. Michelle's. She gets up and goes to bathroom and then gets ready in another bedroom, to try to allow me a short kip or lie-in.

06:35 – I listen to Radio 4 on the BBC iPlayer app on my phone. Despite the interesting news of the weather's impact on agricultural production, I'm still trying to get back to sleep when …

07:00 – My alarm goes off. At the same time, Michelle comes back in with a cup of tea for me. Drink some tea then go to bathroom to ablute.

07:10 – Sit up in bed finishing tea and chatting with Michelle while watching TV breakfast news. I miss most of this news while ranting about Piers Morgan's arrogant, egotistical and manipulative presenting and interview technique. (He has since left that particular employment.)

07:25 – Get fully dressed. Go downstairs. Sometimes pick up bag containing sandwich very kindly prepared for me by Michelle.

07:30 – Get in car. Turn on engine.

07:31 – Get out of car, scrape ice off windscreen.

07:32 – Get back in car and set off.

08:10 – Arrive at car park. Park. Walk to work.

08:15 – Turn computer on. Try to start consultation software. Phone admin staff to ask why consultation software won't start, to be informed that somebody in the building did not turn the computer off last night so necessary downloads and upgrades did not occur. Solutions vary but may include changing password or dialling up technical support helpline or just waiting a few hours until technical support can log in or drive to surgery to sort out problem.

08:20 – If able to access consultation software, start looking at blood test results and newly scanned hospital letters or investigation results.

08:28 – Run upstairs and make a coffee. Walk into admin area and say hi to everyone. See who is off ill.

08:30 – Start three-hour booked surgery – mostly face to face with a few telephone slots. Always run late, especially if interrupted by urgent phone calls from district nurses, hospital doctors, Macmillan nurses, social workers or community psychiatric nurses. (Many surgeries would now expect GPs to do home visits at this stage, but we took turns to do a visit morning or included these on duty days – see chapter end for details.)

12:15 – Look at rest of blood tests and hospital letters. Ring back patients or send messages or emails to staff members to arrange follow-ups or appointments.

13:00 – Go upstairs and make a coffee. Listen to and join in gripes of any other doctors or nurses about their morning lists while there. Bring coffee back downstairs and drink it while eating butty (sandwich) and continuing my trawl through blood and test results and letters.

13:30 – Dictate referral letters or complete online proformas for hospital and investigation referrals.

14:00 – Sign Electronic Prescription Service (EPS) scripts for patients. Also deal with other prescription requests sent by receptionists or practice pharmacist. Mostly, in practice, these are done by the duty doctor.

15:00 – Start three-hour surgery depending on rota. On some days, the afternoon surgery would have a 2 p.m. start and consequently, earlier finish.

18:45 – Finish surgery.

18:45 – Do any urgent referrals. Check blood and other test results and hospital letters.

19:00 – Finish. Walk to car. Drive home.

19:30 – Arrive home.

• • •

Visiting doctor day
Similar to above Standard Day diary, except:

09:00–12:00 – Dealing with all requests for home visits booked or phoned in for that day. Many visit requests can actually be dealt with by a telephone consultation followed by appropriate prescriptions or referrals to other agents. The number of visit requests can vary from zero (this only happened once ever, when I was the visiting doctor) to eighteen.

Aim to actually set off from the surgery at around 11:00 in order to do all the required visits before afternoon duties, although extra visit requests often phoned through after leaving the surgery.

12:00–14:30 – Finish visits, depending on the number and sheer complexity of the visits. The 14:30 finish can be fairly problematic, especially if you are doing a 14:00 surgery. It never looks good to the patients who are sat in the waiting room when the GP wanders in, apparently care-free, half an hour later than your appointment.

· · ·

Duty doctor day

Similar to the above Standard Day diary extract but with the following differences:

09:00 – Three-hour urgent surgery, plus extras. Many more phone call interruptions than when on a routine surgery.

13:00 – Do all of the paperwork as listed earlier plus 1–2 hours of EPS and other prescriptions. Dictate and arrange urgent referrals.

Most days, probably also look online at travel websites, dreaming of, and occasionally booking, holidays.

15:30 – Evening urgent surgery, with extras.

18:30 – Ring several patients back, who have rung with urgent requests during surgery. Very often patients with real or perceived mental health illnesses. Often drunk or otherwise inebriated (the patients, that is, not the GP. Not yet, at least).

Finish off EPS/prescription requests.

Also throughout the day – deal with any urgent visit requests and actual visits, which come in until 18:30. These may all have to be done after 19:30.

The number of late visits done by the GPs has fallen over the past few years as the practice's advanced nurse practitioners (ANPs) have several hours blocked out in order to triage and then do many of the necessary urgent afternoon visits.

In addition to the aforementioned tasks, there are often practice or other meetings to fit in as well as regular training and tutorial sessions for registrars or F2 doctors or students. All of the GPs also provide cover for the trainee doctors, who often need to speak to the GP or request one to come and see their patients with them.

Picture This

Patient, Lyndsey, attending for her consultation but thrusting a smartphone towards me with a blurred photograph on – 'Can you have a look at that photo? It's my husband. He's away working in London and I'm really worried about him.'

Me, ignoring the photograph for a moment, while I tried to find out a bit more – 'Why, what's wrong with him?'

Lyndsey – 'He thinks he's got meningitis.'

Me – 'Gosh, that's a bit worrying. Does he feel very ill?'

Lyndsey – 'No, he doesn't feel ill at all really, but he's got this rash.' Phone again, waving towards me.

Me, pausing, wondering if I should suggest ringing an emergency ambulance for him – 'How long has he had the rash?'

Lyndsey, with completely straight face – 'Six weeks.'

Me, relieved but bemused – 'He's not got meningitis.'

Lyndsey – 'How do you know? You've not even looked at the photo properly.'

Me – 'Because he's had it six weeks.'

Lyndsey – 'But he's looked on Google.'

Me, firmly, for me – 'He has not had meningitis for six weeks.'

Lyndsey – 'Will you look at the photo?'

Me – 'Of course.'

I looked.

Properly.

The photo showed a few dark-red spots on his chest, belly and upper arms. They looked like Campbell de Morgan spots, which are benign (safe, non-serious) skin lesions that anyone can develop, especially if over forty. I explained this to Lyndsey and asked her – 'Are you sure he has only had them six weeks?'

Lyndsey – 'Welllll. I think he's had a few of these for a bit longer than that, but you know what men are like. And you can't be too careful.'

Me – 'Welllll, you probably can, but I understand what you mean. Don't worry. He has not got meningitis.'

Lyndsey – 'OK. I'll just text him to tell him and we can get on with my stuff then.'

She did, and then we did.

Searching for Health

There is nothing wrong with searching the internet for help with understanding health problems. Doctors do it, hopefully to remember long-forgotten syndromes or spellings rather than for spot-the-diagnosis. They would hopefully also tend to use more reputable sites and avoid the larger number of nutty, agenda-driven sites selling useless pseudo-vitamins and pseudo-science.

The other main problem with inputting your symptoms into a search engine is that this tends to tell you what you might have, but never tells you what you don't have, as negative symptoms or indicators are not listed. For example, one particular patient told me they had searched their symptoms on the web and now wondered if they had prostate cancer. I explained that this was unlikely, partly because of the patient's youth (age twenty-three), but mostly because the patient was a woman (with no history of previous sex transition procedures, of course).

Younger patients frequently presented with potential self-diagnoses from the internet, more specifically from social media sites. Most weeks I saw at least one teenager who thought that they had a bipolar mental health condition (often previously known as manic depression). This was usually based on the observation that they (and most of their friends) sometimes felt happy and sometimes sad, on the same day, ergo they must have bipolar disease. An attempted explanation from me about the normality of normal people having different moods and feelings without this being evidence of any disease was often met with sullen disbelief, even after a thorough discussion of their symptoms and mood. On several occasions, I was told that, 'Doctors don't know everything,' often followed by, 'My friends were told the same thing by their doctors, too.'

Similarly, attention deficit hyperactivity disorder (ADHD), autism and dyslexia were very frequently self-presented by adults or by family members for children, of course. The likelihood of these being true diagnoses was much higher than with the self-diagnosis of bipolar disease, but still not usually likely to be accurate on every occasion.

Many struggling mums brought in their brood of unruly youngsters, telling me that they thought that every one of them had at least one of these three conditions, and felt themselves caught up in a battle with the children's nurseries and schools, who were meant to investigate possible cases of these diseases, together with the associated learning difficulties. The schools should offer educational psychology assessments of all children with suspected learning or behavioural problems but would sometimes deflect parents and their offspring to the GP, especially if they had no strong suspicions of their own but were being pressured by parents. Unfortunately, the child psychology services we had access to did not offer educational assessments on demand as they were not funded for this, so we could not refer there either. Many parents felt caught in a trap and bounced between the schools and GPs, looking for an answer to their concerns. Sometimes the parents, if they could afford it, saw a private child educational psychologist, who usually furnished them with confirmation of their suspected diagnosis. This did not always help as much as the families had hoped, because the schools would not usually change their systems to accommodate this, paid-for, opinion. In fairness, many of these presented children had no inbuilt conditions and struggled more because they were being brought up in chaotic, unstructured households. It helped greatly, though, if they had an officially diagnosed condition, as the school could then put in extra support to help these children develop and not be left behind their peers, so the pressure to produce one is understandable.

Violet

Patients, of course, have their own perspective on some absurdities of medical practice. One such patient was my aunt Violet. She started work at fourteen, on the production line at a Trafford Park factory, and after that spent most of her working life as a 'clippy' (female bus conductor or conductress). Unfortunately, her health was poor and she spent quite a lot of her retirement attending her GP surgery and a variety of hospital clinics and wards. She was not impressed by pompous authority and particularly disliked being patronised.

She attended an asthma clinic at her surgery and was at first upset, and then amused, to find that it was upstairs. She, and all of the other clinic attendees, were too breathless, at first, to book in after struggling up the stairs or even undertake the required breathing tests for a while. She suffered from COPD and was at the severe end of the disease spectrum. I pointed out to her that most patients at the clinic would be able to manage a flight of stairs better than she could as they would most likely have better exercise tolerance.

'They shouldn't have put me in that clinic, then,' she answered, probably correctly.

Another clinic, this time at her local hospital. This one was a Hearing Assessment Clinic for the presumed hard-of-hearing, prior to the fitting and provision of hearing aids. It was also upstairs, but at least there was a lift this time. Violet booked in and sat down in the crowded waiting room. A shy young audiologist popped into the waiting room and spoke in a whisper. She looked around the room. No response. She went back into the office. The patients in the waiting room turned to each other and mostly said, 'What did she say?'

The general consensus was that she had called out a patient's name, but none of them had heard which it was. The audiologist came back out of her office and tried again twice more, with no success. Finally, an older, and bolder, audiologist appeared and bellowed out a name. This time the requested patient stood up and said, loudly, 'That's me!'

There was a cheer from the rest of the patients in the waiting room. The same audiologist was sent out every time thereafter that morning.

Violet spent a good while as an inpatient during one particular episode of illness and was noted by the nurses to eat very little of the hospital meals. It was no great matter to her family as we were able to visit her on most days, between us, and bring her favourite M&S sandwiches and snacks. The nurses, though, were keen to try to help her and the other patients who left much of their food, too. She was asked why she did not eat the food, and she replied that the food was generally dreadful, and specifically, cold.

The ward sister said, 'I wish you would complain, as they don't listen to us.'

Violet requested that the head chef come and see her. They did and he did. He was a large, bearded chap wearing his kitchen uniform.

He spoke to Violet. 'They tell me that you want to speak to me about the food.'

'Are you the head chef?' she asked.

'Yes.'

'Well, you're getting money under false pretences,' she said, and then went on to point out the faults that she had found in the food and presentation.

He told her why she was wrong and that it was hard to get hot food to all the patients in the hospital. She pushed back and said that the hot meals should at least arrive hot, otherwise it was a waste of all of their efforts and ingredients. He agreed to see what they could do.

The food improved very quickly after this meeting and started to arrive in powered, heated trolleys, which made a lot of difference. The nurses thanked her as they now found mealtimes a lot more useful and less stressful. The chef popped back to see if Violet was any happier. She was, and told him he could now justify putting his chef's hat and badge back on again.

She was a very determined lady. She spent over four months in hospital on that occasion and was discharged to a nursing home. Her social worker pushed her to give up her rented flat for somebody else, but she was determined to go back to her home and eventually she did. She was happy there and spent much of her time looking at the world passing by outside her window or watching snooker on TV while eating her beloved M&S food.

Ramadan

One of my roles was as a GP trainer. The application process for this involved attending a number of training courses and submitting some written work, which included plans for how the practice would adapt to becoming a suitable training space. It had previously been one until the GP partner who was a trainer had stepped back from this a few years before his retirement. It was generally regarded as a good thing to become a certified training environment; apart from a bit of pride in achieving the standards required, training practices were excused from annual quality inspections for a while.

Trainees, or registrars, were usually allocated to us on a twelve-month placement to complete their GP training. They had already done five or six years at a university medical school, followed by four years working in hospital placements, prior to joining us. Some of these roles and timings changed over the following years, but that is how things were initially.

We seemed to be very lucky with the registrars placed with us. We only had a few who needed a lot of support and encouragement: most were excellent, some were outstanding. One of the latter was Masud. He had been born and brought up in the UK and, to be brutally honest, was not a devout Muslim; no doubt this was in part owing to his mum being a Catholic.

At the time he was our registrar, it was a requirement for registrars to record a number of consultations on video and to submit the best of these as part of their final GP examinations. The patients had to give their consent to the videos being shared for this purpose or for other training purposes. I watched many of these videos with him for analysis of his consultation technique and to help decide on the suitability of videos for exam submission.

One video featured a young Asian lad who had been brought in by his dad because of the lad's earache. The consultation went well and, towards the end, Masud had leant over to examine the boy's ear. The father, who was in traditional dress, took that opportunity to have a good look around the consulting room. He took in the video camera and then his gaze fixed on the coffee cup in front of Masud.

'Brother,' said the father, 'are you a Muslim?'

'Yeah,' said Masud half-heartedly, briefly distracted from his examination.

'Do you practice?' said the dad.

'Yeah, mostly,' said Masud.

'What about Ramadan, brother?'

'Yeah, of course. When is it?' replied Masud, now leaning back from the boy.

'Now!' said the dad firmly, eyes again fixed on the cup of coffee. He then looked at the camera and then at Masud.

There was a long pause. Masud smiled weakly and then continued with the rest of the consultation. By this time I was laughing so much that I was incapable of giving any proper feedback about the consultation (which was excellent, as usual).

In the Country

Our urban practice had a catchment area that was wide enough to encompass several other small towns, as well as a few suburbs and a bit of countryside. We had quite a wide variety of patients: many from very deprived areas, some from the suburban and greener areas. Quite good to have a mixture and variety of folk and professions, although the patients from the more deprived areas tended to attend more often and require more help than the others. A simple example of that would be a patient off work in need of, say, a knee operation. This might require quite a few GP visits for the referral, sick notes and painkillers while waiting for the hospital appointment and then even longer for the operation. In more upmarket areas, in which many patients have private healthcare insurance, they may only attend the surgery once for a private referral and may not need to see the GP again about the knee problem.

Working as a GP in a wealthier area can have its own demands, too. Some well-educated patients can have very specific expectations and demands of the health service, which may be very unrealistic and often wrong. But overall there does seem to be less demand on appointments in those areas, often freeing up GPs to perform other lucrative work outside the practice.

I bumped into a former colleague, Richard, at a GP training event a few years ago. He had worked at a next-door surgery but retired some three years before.

I said, 'What are you doing here? I thought you'd retired?'

Richard replied, 'I did and was glad to get out of the rat race, but one of my friends asked if I could do a few part-time sessions at a surgery near my house.' (In a lovely village on the border between Cheshire and the Peak District.)

I asked him, 'And how is that going?'

Richard replied, 'Oh, I love it. It's nothing like the old prac-tice. In fact, it's not like work at all. No stress. No aggro. It's really different from being in a town. I did a surgery yesterday and the only problem I had was waiting for my last patient. She turned up late as she had to round up her horse before she rode it to the surgery.'

'You are joking?' I asked, laughing now.

'No. She tied it up outside the surgery. There's a metal ring thingy on the wall.'

I replied, 'If they tied a horse up outside our surgery, it would be on bricks when they came out and somebody would have nicked the horseshoes.'

'And it would have been a Motability horse anyway,' said Richard.

Conversion

I am an atheist despite – or maybe because of – attending a Catholic grammar school from the age of eleven: taught mostly by Christian Brothers. I could never grasp the faith, despite my keen efforts. Many years later, my mother was shocked to find out, from Michelle, that I believed myself to be an atheist and quickly corrected her with, 'Well, he's a Catholic atheist, then!'

I was always careful at work to show respect for patients' beliefs, religious or not. Actually, in the spirit of full and open disclosure, I did take the mickey out of my Catholic GP colleagues, feeling that was OK, as I had dipped my toe in that particular holy water a bit. I would not dream of attempting such humour with my colleagues of other faiths.

Of course, people have all sorts of non-formal beliefs that can offer support as well. I tried to explore these belief systems – formal, non-formal or family – with patients when considering their support systems and networks. I would always keep my beliefs to myself, unless asked. This attitude was not shared by some of my patients and even colleagues. Several Muslim patients, and one registrar, were keen, and with kind intention, to push me towards Islamic studies and possible conversion. I was given numerous books about this faith. The registrar, additionally, gave me as a leaving gift a book decrying Western science, with special focus on the 'myth' of evolution. I remained unswayed in my non-belief.

A Mormon minister gave me several copies of *The Book of Mormon** over the years. Towards the end of every consultation

---

* Before the famous musical show of the same name, which I later went to see in London. The minister was unimpressed by my non-biblical revelation of that trip.

he would ask me how my reading and understanding of the book was going. I would usually try to deflect his questioning with (to my mind) humour.

'It's come in really handy, as one of our tables at home was a bit wobbly and the book has levelled it up.'

His response: 'We'll get you in the end. We always do.'

I thanked him for his interest and kindness but told him that he was wasting his time, and mine, to some extent.

'You are a really good doctor and a good man, and I want to save you on the Day of Reckoning. Which is very near, as you would realise if you read the book.'

He passed away a few years ago. I hope that his faith was a comfort to him and his family.

Welcome

One duty day I was called to visit a woman in her early twenties who was suffering from abdominal pain and felt unable to get to the surgery. I parked up near the small block of flats she lived in, walked up to the second floor and knocked. A dog barked loudly from within; the noise had started as I was walking up the stairs two floors below. A tall, broad man answered the door, barely managing to keep a large, salivating dog – exuding muscle and pure rage – under control via a thick metal chain.

'Is it the doctor? Are you lookin' for Tracy?' he shouted.

'Yes!'

'Come in, she's in 'ere. Don't worry, I won't let Max get yer,' he added, still shouting.

I was grateful that he would ensure that I wouldn't be attacked by his dog. He stood back in the hallway as I squeezed past against the opposite wall, while Max strained every sinew trying to reach me. Thankfully for me, he didn't manage and I went into the living room.

Tracy was lying on her side on the sofa, her head propped by her arm up on the sofa arm. I walked towards her and perched myself on a pouffe in front of her after asking if that was OK. She'd grunted her assent.

Her partner sat down in an armchair behind me. Max had stopped barking by then, although I could still feel his breath on the nape of my neck. I started to ask Tracy about her symptoms, conscious of the dog and also, now, the loud TV to my right side. Tracy did not seem to be concentrating or listening to my questions. She was also trying to look around me at the TV. I looked over my shoulder to see what was so important: it was *The Jeremy Kyle Show*.

I asked, 'Can you turn the telly off, please?'

Tracy replied, 'I'll just turn it down a bit,' and did.

I continued. Tracy also continued to look distracted and irritated by my questions and then also propped herself up to look over my head at the TV while I knelt down to examine her abdomen.

'I can't examine you while you are watching this. Please turn it off,' I tried again.

'No, 'cos my mate's on it in a minute,' she said.

It was clear by now that she was not very ill and more interested in watching the programme than talking to me. I told her to book an appointment at the surgery so that she could be examined properly. She didn't seem that bothered and turned the TV back up before I had even left the room. Max took his cue and returned to his previous role and volume as he escorted me through the doorway onto the landing, just as a pizza delivery arrived.

Bad News

As a doctor, you are only one letter or phone call away from a complaint or being sued, or even being struck off. You might think that a doctor can prevent any such worry by just being very good and careful and thorough, but I think that the days when just being a 'good' doctor can immunise you against such actions have long gone. Complaints against GPs and their surgeries are often over the most trivial things or about things that are completely outside their control. I am not against patients having the right to complain or sue; my family and I are also patients and have had many reasons to be concerned about the level of care at times, and about the actions and explanations of staff at others.

There are times when the GPs or nurses in a practice can look back on the care of an individual patient with regret and wonder if things could have been done better. Certainly, any time there is a near miss or actual incident identified then the practice and relevant team members will arrange a critical incident review, which concludes with changes in practices and processes to try to help minimise the risk of such incidents recurring in the future.

Many phoned-in or written complaints are successfully defused by the practice manager who, certainly in our case, is skilled at mediating, and also not frightened of telling the GPs off if she thinks there is any element of blame or lack of care. Probably the largest number of complaints in most surgeries is the inability of patients to book a GP appointment with their GP of choice when they want it. This problem worsened during the pandemic.

Many other complaints usually involve cases in which numerous GPs and/or hospital doctors have been involved, with the associated increased potential for miscommunications, and failed referrals for further investigations and treatments. These often take a long time to address and sort out due to the sheer numbers of people involved and their differing interpretations and reports of events.

If there is a failure of mediation and patients or their relatives are still keen to make a complaint then they will often deal with responsible ombudsman, or even go directly to a solicitor or the General Medical Council (GMC) itself. At this stage, or even earlier, it is also often wise for the GP to speak with their medical defence insurers, who can give support and advice. Until recently the cost of this insurance was greater than £10,000 a year for each GP, but fortunately the government is gradually taking over the responsibility for this insurance. They had previously already taken on the insurance costs for hospital doctors many years ago.

The first time I had to deal with a complaint and also involve my insurers was while I was still a GP registrar working in my GP training post. This complaint was in regard to a patient I had been called to see one morning at 6.30 a.m. She was an elderly lady who had chest pain and in those days the first port of call was still the GP rather than the ambulance service. The lady was distressed and breathless and also had an apparent deep-vein thrombosis (DVT). I felt that she most likely had a pulmonary embolism (PE), secondary to her DVT, and I arranged for an emergency ambulance to take her to the local hospital A&E unit. I stayed with her until the crew arrived and helped to stabilise her for transfer. She could barely speak, but the oxygen they gave her at least helped her levels of distress. I then drove to the surgery and filled in the details on her records.

The first I heard from my medical indemnity insurers was a claim against me for admitting this lady without referring to an allergy that she had to an antibiotic drug called Septrin. It appeared that she was administered this while in hospital and had become rather ill as a consequence. She had developed a nasty condition called Stevens-Johnson syndrome: a reaction characterised by widespread sores on the body and ulcers in the mouth and eyes. Septrin was known to be one of the causal factors for this condition. She had recovered but had suffered greatly during her hospital stay.

I was shocked and upset to be confronted by a claim against me when I had done my best in such an emergency situation. The claim included suggestions that I was her GP and that I had access to her records, which would have had reference to her known drug allergies, and I should have included these details on the letter I sent with her to hospital. My defence against this claim was focused on the fact that I had not had access to this lady's records when I saw her and nor had I been able to gain a very good history from her as she was so breathless. I would also not have expected use of this drug for a suspected PE even if I had known about this allergy.

My other defence came from my knowledge of this lady's admission from another source – her daughter. Her daughter was a patient at the same practice. She had also told me how distressed she and her family had been while her mum was in hospital. She told me about their fury at her mum being given Septrin, despite repeatedly and pointedly informing the medical and nursing staff on at least three occasions that she was allergic to it.

I spoke to an advisor at my medical my insurers and also gave them the required written response. I told them about the other information I had heard from the lady's family. The insurers found out that it was the hospital's lawyers who were trying to switch the blame to me in order to reduce or minimise the hospital's culpability. The case was eventually settled by the hospital.

The daughter later told me that she and the family had been stunned by the hospital's attempt to switch blame and were glad that things had been sorted out more fairly.

Many years later, one of my GP colleagues, Norman, was involved in a prolonged case, which, after five years, reached the High Court in London. Ten days before the hearing, it was decided that I may also have had some involvement in the case, as I had been on duty on the day that the patient first fell ill, so I was required to write a statement and also attend court to read it. Norman and I travelled down to London by train on the Sunday and he was able to fill me in on the details of the case, which hinged on claims that we, as a practice, had delayed the admission of a patient who'd had a stroke and that the alleged delay had had a negative effect on his outcome.

Early on the Monday morning we met up with the defence lawyer in the court chambers in the Temple area off Fleet Street, later being joined by our barrister, who parked his beautiful Aston Martin by the office window. Later still, we were joined by our medical expert, an eminent and renowned neurosurgeon, who was very helpful and reassuring about the case. An hour or so later we left the office together and walked to the High Court, arriving there via the famous zebra crossing, which often features on news bulletins, as news photographers usually stand over the other side of the road, snapping litigants emerging from the High Court onto said crossing. Uncomfortable and embarrassed, we also nearly bumped into our accusers as we walked through the court lobby on the way to the courtroom. In the end, the hearing only lasted for a few sessions, the defence case being greatly aided by the neurosurgeon, who was also the author of some of the articles referred to by the litigants in their case. We were found not to have neglected our duty of care for the patient in any way. We had presumed this, but attending court was still a very stressful event.

Two weeks later, I saw the patient in the surgery about his usual medical problems. Afterwards, he spoke to me in a whisper. 'Sorry about the court thing. It was never personal, but things are tough for us, as you know, so the money would have come in handy.'

'Of course. I understand,' I said, surprisingly meaning it, as I did feel sorry for him and his wife, who also had significant health problems. They stayed as patients at our surgery until they moved outside our catchment area five years later.

Bedtime Drink

Moira was a ninety-year-old patient, well known to the surgery staff for her neediness and her demands for regular reviews and emergency appointments. She appeared remarkably fit for her age, but she did not agree with that assessment. She lived alone and still drove. She seemed to have little contact with her children. Her attention-seeking behaviour may have been caused by her loneliness or even been the cause of it. Most weeks she obtained at least one urgent appointment, and at most of these she was stripping off and heading to the examination couch before even sitting down.

At one of these urgent slots she told me that she had spent most of the night at A&E and had been told to go and see her GP urgently.

Me – 'Why, what happened?'

Moira – 'I was thirsty last night when I was in bed. I reached over to grab my glass of water from my bedside table. I drank it all then realised it was a bottle of calamine lotion that I'd drunk.'

I laughed.

'What, a full bottle before you realised it wasn't water?'

Moira, frowning at me – 'Yes. It wasn't a big bottle.'

Me – 'You must have realised it wasn't a glass when you unscrewed the lid?'

Moira – 'No. It was dark.'

I started laughing again at this point and found it very difficult to stop.

Moira – 'Well, I'm surprised at you, of all people. I thought you were kind. They were really worried about me in A&E and told me you might need to do some blood tests. Or something. They insisted.'

I doubted that they had actually insisted she get an urgent GP appointment and it was more likely she had used her A&E attendance as a ticket to get another appointment with us. I amused myself wondering whether there was a calamine lotion blood test available, but before I got too smug, Moira had already got up and was heading towards the examination couch.

She had stripped off, fully, before I had even managed to close the curtains around the couch.

'I thought you might want to examine me, doctor, just to make sure I haven't come to any harm. You owe me that after laughing at me.'

Oh, bugger.

I rang through to reception for a chaperone, aware that it would now take even longer to get her to leave the room, hopefully for at least another week this time.

Why Has General Practice Changed?

Most patients with chronic long-term medical conditions are now managed entirely at their GP surgery, which is very different from when I started in practice. At that time, it seemed that the only chronic disease managed fully by GPs was hypertension (high blood pressure), with diabetic care being shared with medical consultants in hospital.

As well as this change, the actual number of people living with chronic disease seems to have increased across the board. There is no evidence that people are actually any more sick than they were then, so perhaps we are now more aware of such illnesses. Also, as treatments become more effective and available, people naturally come forward to seek access: these treatments including, for instance, hip and knee joint replacements and cataract surgery.

We also treat many more conditions in a preventative manner than we did then, such as high cholesterol and pre-diabetes. Many of these require regular blood tests and reviews. Patients therefore have many more reasons to attend the surgery than they did in the past, when the chief reason for booking an appointment at the GP's was feeling acutely unwell, or finding a new lump or symptom. Patients are also required to attend for vaccinations and for contraception, of course, and have generally higher expectations of their bodies overall, and of the NHS in helping to manage them.

Many patients therefore have more reasons than ever to attend the GP surgery, apart from feeling ill, only to find that many more other patients have also done the same. The number of appointments offered, and taken, per patient per year is a lot higher than it was, but this is still not enough. Demand was high even before the Covid pandemic and appears to be even higher now, according to the medical press and confirmed by the doctors in my old practice. The supposed reason for this increase is deemed to be the large number of patients who put off attending their GP during lockdown, but who are now trying to sort out the issues that they deferred. In addition to this, all of the current and growing delays in planned hospital investigations and treatments mean that those waiting need more GP treatment and support in the meantime.

By the time patients get in for their appointment, they have often developed a long list of problems and worries to discuss. Appointment times have increased in most practices to allow for these changes, but this still often does not feel long enough. When I started at my practice, appointments were usually for five minutes and are now usually fifteen minutes long, and yet are still more likely to run late now than they were in the 1980s.

Overall, working hours for GPs and other doctors in this country are far lower and better than they used to be, but are often reported as feeling more difficult and stressful. As stated already, I think that patients' expectations and demands are higher and this adds to the perceived burden. The younger doctors have nothing to compare their workload with and maybe the older ones, myself included, have forgotten how things once were. The modern-day workload remains mentally and emotionally draining, however, especially if you invest yourself personally in the care and support you offer patients.

'Is There a Doctor on Board?'

I was on an Air China flight from Bangkok to Amsterdam. About four hours into the flight, I was just drifting off to sleep while watching a film. The announcement jolted me awake.

'Is there a doctor on board?'

I told the stewardess that I was a doctor. She led me quickly to a lady in another part of the plane. This lady had passed out and had become unrousable, and her husband had quickly alerted the staff. The lady was Dutch and in her fifties. I thought it best to lay her down quickly in the aisle for better assessment and for CPR if needed, and one of the stewardesses fetched the emergency medical kit.

The Dutch lady was still breathing, had a clear airway and a reasonable pulse, but a very low blood pressure. Her husband was worried that she may have had a stroke as her mother had previously suffered one. I gave her oxygen initially and she started to come around, although was a bit groggy. There were no obvious signs of a stroke. At this stage I thought we should move her to a business class seat if there were any free; she could be laid flat and there would be more space around for assessment and any treatment that may become necessary. They found two such empty seats and we carried this lady to one, and her husband joined her in the next seat.

The lady was speaking a bit more coherently by now and reported no symptoms before her faint, nor any currently, apart from just feeling a bit weak. By this time the co-pilot had come back to check how things were and seemed extremely relieved to find that I did not think we needed to divert the plane for an early landing. I said I would need to keep popping back from cattle class to check on this lady, and the stewardesses agreed. I looked enviously and hopefully at the other empty business seats in this cabin of the plane, but this elicited no response.

I tried again a little more directly. 'It might be better if I stayed in one of these seats in order to keep an eye on her.'

The stewardess smiled and said, 'No. Is fine. You come and see lady, and we come and get you if we need you.'

I went back to my seat and slept fitfully, popping back to see the Dutch lady a few times. She was much better as we approached landing. I suggested that she was assessed by the airport medical staff, but she was keener to get home and see her own doctor later that day. She and her husband thanked me.

The head steward and stewardess handed me a bottle of Moët champagne in a sealed, tamper-proof customs bag, together with an explanatory letter for the security staff at Schiphol Airport, asking them not to confiscate the bottle.

I disembarked and headed through security towards the next gate and flight. I handed the letter and bottle to a security staff member by the conveyor belt and X-ray machine. I explained what the letter was about. He gave me a lopsided smile and while holding constant eye contact with me, tore the letter into shreds. He then lifted the Moët bottle to head height and dropped it from there into the liquids bin, saying, 'Thank you, sir. Next!'

The second occasion was in winter, on a Lufthansa jumbo-jet flight from Frankfurt to Vancouver, Canada.

'Can any doctors on the flight please make themselves known to the chief stewardess at the bottom of the stairs.'

I was keen to help, not having been asleep this time. I went quickly to the stairs. There was quite a crowd of people there already, for some reason.

The chief stewardess was also there and shouted, 'Doctors only here, please.'

Nobody moved.

She spoke more quietly this time. 'Are you all doctors?'

We all nodded. She then asked what exactly we all did (speaking in excellent English, of course). It was a roll call of emergency medical hierarchy. Everyone answered in English, even the German doctors, speaking to the German stewardess on the German airline. The list included an anaesthetist, an A&E consultant and a cardiologist. These three were selected, probably most appropriately, and the rest of us were told that we could sit back down. Another stewardess who was stood with us said, 'It's no wonder you can never get a doctor in Europe. You're all going skiing.'

That appeared to be the case, certainly for me. I sat back down with my friend and travelling ski partner, Mick, who was also a doctor. In his case a 'real doctor' with proper academic qualifications, rather than the courtesy title that medical doctors are given. In fairness, he would also have been able to help in many medical emergencies due to him also having mountain leadership experience, with the associated first-aid training that he had received. Thankfully, there were no further calls on my medical, nor on Mick's academic or emergency skills during that flight.

An hour later, a stewardess came over to us and offered us bonus drinks in appreciation. These drinks were not confiscated. They would have had to be quick.

Lists

It is often said, especially on TV or radio programmes, that patients should bring a written list so that they don't forget to mention something important when they attend a GP appointment. This seems sensible, especially if patients are forgetful. It seems reasonable that they might need to mention a few symptoms and areas of concern during a consultation, and also reasonable to discuss a hospital referral or prescription request. Lots of patients have more than one medical condition and consultations can often therefore be complex, so a written reminder useful for this. Helpful and sensible to have a list! What could possibly go wrong?

Unfortunately, some patients don't know when to stop. It is very common for patients to attend with a seven- or eight-problem list and it is not at all unusual for GPs to be faced with a twenty-line list or even more. It is extremely difficult for a doctor to try to help with such lists in a single consultation, although they often try, as they are sympathetic and realise it is difficult to arrange further appointments. GP appointments often overrun because of this and it unfair on the GP and unfair on the other patients who are waiting. Some GPs and some surgeries now have a 'one problem per consultation' rule to try to cope with this, with related posters in the waiting room and on GP doors.

We resisted this at my practice as we viewed it as petty and antagonistic, and besides, a single disease can itself cause several symptoms or problems. I wrote a short article for our practice newsletter asking patients to moderate their lists. It had no impact whatsoever, of course.

One way of trying to cope with lists was for us to have a List of the Week award as entertainment at our weekly GP meetings. These regularly featured full-page A4 lists. I won once with a two-and-a-half A4 page list of closely written text. The patient had also added, verbally, during the consultation, and after I had scanned through this list:

'The other thing, that I really came in with, is …' and proceeded to ask me about two other significant concerns, and then to ask me to do a referral for her dad and prescriptions for her two children. And then asked how her husband's scan result had been. Saying, 'No,' takes time, especially when trying to be polite, but she persisted long enough to get angry with me for only tackling the key problems on her written list and two of her significant bonus items.

My colleague, Masud, once won with a fantastic illustration that a patient had brought in. This picture would happily grace a textbook. It was a colour drawing of a person, with arrows pointing to twenty or so different areas of the patient's anatomy, with speech bubbles listing the problems and symptoms relating to that area. It was a work of art. Masud had been impressed enough to attempt to review most of the items on the list. In the end, the patient was furious that he had only dealt with the first seventeen of the problems at this one consultation and made a written complaint. It was a shame that the complaint was not done in pictorial form, too.

Humour apart, it still amazed me after many years that even young people could bring in such very long written lists of problems, often with bonus extra verbal problems. These patients often came in every week or so and it probably goes without saying that these patients were usually not very ill. Some were cyberchondriacs, turning up with printouts from their intense internet searches. Their weekly lists often contained more health concerns that had apparently developed in a week than most of us develop in a lifetime. Perhaps the practice needs to revisit the 'one problem' rule.

My former GP trainer, Bill, thought it was a good idea to grab hold of the patient's list, in order to retain control of the consultation. Not just grab in an intellectual sense, but physically get hold of the actual written paper list, if this existed. He told me this on one of the few occasions I actually sat in with him, in order to observe his morning surgery and consultation style. We were sitting in one of the branch surgeries in a village a few miles away from the main surgery. Before calling in a lady in her eighties, Beattie, he turned to me and told me that she always brought a list in, and that he would take it off her and take control of the consultation. He called Beattie from the doorway of the consulting room and in she came. He introduced Beattie and I to each other and we both smiled and nodded. Beattie perched herself on the edge of the chair, handbag on her knee.

There was, as anticipated, paper folded in her left hand.

'Can I just take that, please?' asked Bill, now also nodding and looking over his reading glasses towards the paper that Beattie grasped, now a little tighter. She did not respond.

'Please can I have a look?' he asked, more politely now but leaning forwards.

Beattie leant back slightly now, looking a bit confused, but did not stop him from pulling the paper out of her hand. The paper unscrunched a little to reveal itself as a tissue: obviously already used.

'Oh, sorry. I thought it was for me,' said a blushing Bill as he put the tissue on the desk.

Beattie picked it up and stuffed it up her sleeve, safe for now.

Control of the consultation had been ceded completely to her and she obtained all the diagnoses and referrals and scripts she wanted that morning, with little debate.

After she left the room, Bill turned his chair towards me, shrugged his shoulders and said, 'You can't win 'em all. Shall we get a coffee?'

· · ·

Some examples of (non-award-winning) lists that I have found in my files:

List 1 – it was handwritten, in capitals:

PERMANENT HEADACHE

DIZZINESS/VERTIGO

UNSTEADY ON FEET

LEGS GIVING WAY – CAN'T WALK FAR

NAUSEA

RIBS SWOLLEN

BREATHLESSNESS

EXHAUSTION / NO ENERGY

SLEEP 12–18 HRS (STILL TIRED)

DEPRESSION / BREAKDOWN

NO MOTIVATION TO DO JOBS

DOUBLE VISION (WHEN TIRED)

PANIC ATTACKS

WANT TO TRY LAST BUT ONE ANTIDEPRESSANT TABLET AGAIN. BEGINS WITH D

HEEL PAIN (RT). DIFFERENT TO LAST ONE / PAIN FURTHER BACK

LEFT EAR ITCHING. RIGHT EAR PAIN

WANT RE-REFERRING TO PHYSIO FOR RIGHT KNEE

WANT STEROID INJECTION LEFT SHOULDER AGAIN

NEW STEROID CREAM FOR ECZEMA. FRIEND HAS GOOD ONE IN BLUE TUBE. FEELS GREASY BUT ISN'T

PLEASE HAVE BLOOD TEST VITAMIN B12?

CHEST INFECTION. ANTIBIOTIC

List 2 – also handwritten, in capitals:

1. HEART BYPASS IS SUCCESSFUL. DISCHARGED NOW. MANCHESTER DOCTOR STATED THAT BLOOD CLOT IN LEFT LUNGS WILL BE SUPERVISED BY MY OWN DOCTOR I.E. SCAN, ETC. STILL NO ACTION

2. BOTH SHOULDERS STILL PENDING

3. HERNIA OPERATION IS STILL PENDING

4. I HAVE STARTED SEVERE PAIN IN LEFT RIBS + GOING UPWARDS

5. I WAS TOLD THAT PROBABLY HAVE PROBLEM:
    A – SUGAR; B – KIDNEY; C – BLOOD PRESSURE; D – LIVER?

6. CURRENT SITUATION
    A – ULTRASOUND
    B – BLOOD TEST WAS CARRIED OUT ON 15TH JULY

7. I AM VERY WORRIED ABOUT ONE STONE BODY WEIGHT WITHIN ONE TO ONE AND A HALF MONTHS

8. I WAS PRESCRIBED MACROGOL COMPD — NOT EFFECTIVE. I AM STILL USING? LACTORUS FOUR TIMES A DAY (NOW NO MORE LEFT)

9. HEARING??? — USE OLIVE OIL — SEEMS TO HAVE NO EFFECT, ETC.

10. TUMMY PAIN. UPPER LEFT. WORSE WHEN EATING OR WHEN MISS MEAL. NEW SCAN PLEASE (LAST ONE THREE MONTHS AGO — PAIN DIFFERENT)

11. THAT ONE-A-DAY ANTIBIOTIC. TO KEEP IN CASE GET WATER INFECTION.

12. LETTER FOR REHOUSING / NEIGHBOURS NOISY / DOG

'I Knew You Knew'

One of the heroes of General Practice is Michael Balint,* who helped GPs to look at the psychological dynamics of consultations in a different way. Sometimes the focus was particularly aimed at trying to help with the more complex, difficult or heartsink† patients, for whom it seemed very tricky to crack their real underlying, hidden issues. One of the recognised techniques was the 'flash' (no, not what you are thinking), in which the GP reflected their own feelings back to the patient in the hope of helping them gain some insight into how their problems appeared to others. Some (clever) GPs still meet today in Balint groups to share their experiences and techniques in this regard. Even I often tried to use some of these techniques to try to unlock patients' underlying issues, with occasional success. In truth, however, most of the sudden 'flashes' occurred accidentally, but still helped the mutual understanding of the patient's underlying problems.

---

* A Hungarian-born psychoanalyst who moved to Manchester in 1939. In Britain, he was a main influence for setting up groups for medical doctors to discuss psychological factors in their patients' presentations of illness. These seminars provided opportunities for GPs to discuss with him, and each other, how to understand and help patients. The Balint Society has helped to continue this work since his death in 1970.
† A rather disapproving description of patients who make your heart sink when you see their names on your appointment list. A more thoughtful and understanding approach by some GPs is to say that there are no real heartsink patients, but perhaps heartsink problems or, maybe even, heartsink doctors, who used these labels for patients they were struggling to understand or help.

One of our regular heartsinks was a lady in her mid-seventies, Marjorie. It was a relief to spot her name on somebody else's list rather than your own. This lady was always generally quite miserable and attended with a long list of medical problems. Her agenda was often to try to get the GP to increase and add to the numerous sedatives and antidepressants that she was, or had been, on. The doctor's agenda was usually the opposite. She had also been under the care of a variety of psychiatrists and psychologists over the years. On one occasion, I realised that she had already been on antidepressants and antipsychotic medications before the Beatles had even had their first hit; our chances of completely unravelling all of those years of illness and associated sedation were small. At one point, I mentioned this to her and decided to ask if she had endured a difficult childhood.

'I knew you knew,' she said.

'Knew what?' I asked.

'You know. What happened.'

'I don't really, what are you telling me?' I asked, starting to realise.

She went on to tell me about years of abuse by a close family member, at a time 'before anybody talked about things like that'. The abuser was long gone, but the psychological damage had still impacted on her whole life and being. I can't say that her mental and physical health seemed any better after her revelation, but she frequently mentioned my acknowledgement of her trauma thereafter, and told me that I understood her and felt that I was her friend.

Hannah was cheerful lady of a similar age. I saw her during an afternoon surgery. She had booked an appointment for a shoulder injection. I had already seen her brother on another appointment earlier that afternoon. He was also a cheerful chap, with a farmer's complexion and a jolly smile. He told me that he had just seen his sister in the waiting room and she was seeing me soon.

I mentioned her brother as she sat down in the chair.

A dark cloud passed across her face. 'I don't talk about that man,' she said.

'Oh, sorry, I didn't realise. He seemed quite happy to see you.'

'Well, I'm not happy to see him. I wish he was dead.'

'Sorry to hear that.'

'He was, sorry, is, a horrible brother.'

'Sorry to hear that.'

'He abused me for years. My parents knew all about it. They blamed me and I was made the black sheep of the family, and he was the blue-eyed boy.'

Bloody hell.

It's hard to imagine the pain that some people have had to live with. Hannah appeared to have fared a little bit better than Marjorie, but like her, declined any referral for support or legal action. Also, like Marjorie, she often referred to her revealed trauma in later consultations and told me that I understood her better now.

* * *

David suffered from diabetes and its associated complications. He was a retired classics teacher in his eighties. Several of the receptionists had a soft spot for him as he had taught them at the old local girls' grammar school. I had first got to know him during the many years that he had cared, lovingly, for his wife, Shelly. She had suffered from severe rheumatoid arthritis, but then developed dementia and, finally, terminal breast cancer. David was a devoted husband and struggled for a year or so after he lost her. His mood seemed to lift a bit when he talked about resuming his travels after the many years when he and Shelly had been unable to go very far. He had dusted off his passport and flown out to Athens, Crete and Rome, as befitted a classics scholar. He showed me a few photos during our consultations in between his trips.

'Is it difficult, travelling on your own?' I asked.

'Not too bad, and I sometimes go with a friend, Stephen. In fact, we're off on a trip to Liverpool this weekend. He's going to see Morrissey again and I'm going to try to find an art gallery that stays open a bit later than normal, and then I'll wait for him in a bar till his show is over.'

'Morrissey? Don't you fancy going to see him?' I asked.

'I do not! Absolutely not. He's not my cup of tea. Stephen is a lot younger than me.'

I'm not sure why or what made me say what I said next, apart from my belief that many of Morrissey's fans felt themselves to be disenfranchised or outsiders of sorts. I was not trying to pry or be judgemental.

'Is your friend gay?' I asked.

'I thought you knew,' David said with a broad smile on his face. 'He's gay, and so am I. I have been dying to tell you for ages now.'

'Well, I didn't know,' I said.

'I daren't tell my daughters 'cos they'll go mad, so it's nice that somebody knows. I thought you'd sussed me out.'

'Not really,' I protested.

'I really loved Shelly, you know, and we had a good life together. But now I think I deserve to be me for a bit.'

'You could not have done any more for her, I'm sure,' I said.

'Thank you. I hope so. You were a great help, too.'

A charming man, indeed.

Baby Talk

I had popped round to the reception area and was signing prescriptions and answering queries for the receptionists and pharmacist. I was sitting on a stool in front of a computer, just out of sight of the front desk, talking to one of the receptionists, Sue. While I was there she dealt with a few patients booking appointments and then a young couple came to the desk. They were carrying a small baby.

'Hello,' said the gentleman. 'We have come to register baby.'

He spoke with a strong East European accent.

'OK,' said Sue. 'Can I just take some details?' She proceeded with this task and the couple were able to answer and then provide the required written information, which included looking at the child's birth registration.

Sue then said, 'Language. What's the first language?' A slightly clumsy question, admittedly. There was a considered pause.

The dad then answered, 'We don't know. The baby has not spoken yet. He is six weeks old.'

I whispered to Sue, 'Ask them to guess what language the baby might speak. Chinese, maybe?' She glared at me while scrunching up her lips. The look suggested that I was not being helpful.

Sue tried again, this time with a bit more precision. 'What is the first language in your home?'

'Polish, but we promise we will speak to baby in English as well,' said the dad, keen to help.

'I'll just put Polish, thanks,' said Sue, and completed the registration.

She told me off afterwards as she was already struggling to avoid laughing before I chipped in. It was also a bit rude of me to be whispering jokes out of their earshot, I know, especially as it was the nature of our questions that had led to the Polish chap's honest answer. We later agreed at a GP partner meeting that we should slightly amend the questions for new patient registration in order to make things a bit less confusing.

'You Are Invited to Attend the Inquest'

GPs often fear the in-tray, as I have already mentioned. The arrival of a hospital discharge letter or notification of a hospital death often prompts a quick search of the patient's records to see which GP last saw or dealt with the patient. Partially from curiosity and interest, but also for self-protection. Hoping that nobody has missed anything preventable or treatable. Hoping mostly that it wasn't you.

Another letter that requires a definite response, by law, is a coroner's letter. These usually arrive a few weeks after the unexpected death of a patient, requesting details of their full medical history with a focus on the last twelve months, including all recently prescribed medications. The coroner also, later, declares the date of an inquest and states that the GP may be required to attend on this date. Most often, nearer the time of the inquest, the coroner writes to state that the GP is not required to attend in person and that their written report is enough.

I was required to attend four inquests in person, to read out my statement and answer questions asked by the coroner or family members. These were stressful experiences, not dissimilar to being on trial, especially when the family were angry at the death of their loved one and looking for somebody to blame.

One of the inquests followed a drug overdose by a patient, Graham, with a long history of alcohol and drug usage: prescribed and illicit. The family seemed keen to blame the GPs for prescribing the medications used in the overdose and questioned me at some length. This was a difficult experience for several reasons. Firstly, you do carry a sense of responsibility as a doctor whenever a patient dies, from whatever cause. Secondly, the members of the family had often attended with Graham, begging us to prescribe strong sedative medications to avoid him having to buy any. It was difficult, to be honest: I was conscious that the family had lost somebody they loved and some sensitivity was required even in the face of aggressive questioning. Graham had also been under the care of substance misuse services as well as an NHS, and also a private, psychiatrist. Luckily for me, if not for the deceased and his family, the toxicology reports were revealed near to the end of the inquest and they showed that the drugs implicated in his death were five different, non-prescription, drugs.

The family, afterwards, still came to our surgery as patients and I regularly saw Graham's mum up to my retirement. You have to take the long view and accept the understandable anger and the need to hit out that the bereaved can feel.

I also attended the inquest of a lady in her seventies, Lily. She had died following a severe haemorrhagic stroke: this being a stroke caused by bleeding into the brain, rather than the much more common embolic stroke, which is caused by a clot inside the brain arteries. This poor lady had suffered from atrial fibrillation (AF) and was on treatment with anticoagulants, which are given to minimise the high risk of clots, which AF causes. The especially unfortunate part of this lady's death was that the anticoagulant drug itself was likely to have been the reason that her brain bleed had become so extensive and therefore fatal. The coroner on this occasion effectively used his interview of me in order to help the family understand the sequence of events leading up to Lily's death. The family were angry that the prescribed anticoagulant had led to her death and questioned me in that regard.

The coroner helpfully pointed out that had the GPs not prescribed the anticoagulant then the family were far more likely to have been attending an inquest or trying to sue the GPs for neglect. The family, especially Lily's husband, Sid, were still upset and a bit angry at the end of the inquest. Sid did, however, continue to see me in the surgery for his routine and urgent appointments. He was always friendly, often remembering Lily and also his mum and dad, who had previously been patients of mine.

Nora

I visited Nora, a lovely lady in her upper eighties. I had been her GP for over twenty years but had not seen her for a few years at this point. She now had established dementia and was receiving quite a lot of support at home from family and from paid carers and also district nurses. The district nurses had requested a visit for her as she had also now developed leg ulcers, which were potentially infected and were healing poorly. Her niece was present when I arrived and she let me in. She explained that Nora was a bit confused but generally understood what was going on.

I walked into Nora's living room and found her sitting in the middle of the room in a high-backed armchair.

'Where's Dr S?' she asked.

I replied, 'I am Dr S.'

'No you're not,' she insisted. 'He had hair.'

'I've gone bald,' I said.

'Dr S had a beard,' she said.

'I've shaved my beard off,' I said.

'Dr S wore glasses,' she continued.

'I've had my eyes lasered, so I don't need glasses,' I said, and then added, 'I'm having a sex change tomorrow.'

'Ooh, don't do that, love. You still look handsome as a man.'

'Thank you. I was only teasing you. Sorry.'

'Ooh, I know it's you now, with your cheeky sense of humour,' she chuckled.

The ice was broken and she chatted with me as the old friend she was, joking much of the time as she always used to. I saw her a few more times afterwards, although fairly predictably, but still sadly, her dementia and physical condition deteriorated over the next six months. She passed away in a local nursing home, loved and looked after by family and care staff till the end: still joking with everyone who came in to see her.

Dope

Anybody walking through a UK city centre can see evidence of the effects of drug use on society, and anyone in the police force or NHS has seen and dealt with the more direct and indirect effects on individuals. When working in A&E, I had seen and treated numerous injecting drug addicts who had severely damaged their own veins. Many had used and damaged the usual arm veins so much that they were now unusable for them to inject, hence they looked for ever more unsuitable veins until these also blocked up or became badly infected. Several had needed leg amputations, partial and even full. I also saw two men who had required amputations of their penises after using and damaging the blood vessels there. Pretty desperate, to say the least.

In our practice area, there is a surprisingly large number of relatively young men limping and using walking sticks. I recently counted six of these when I walked into the town centre and recognised every one as an addict who had damaged their own legs due to vein thromboses or infections.

Dope smoking appears endemic in some areas and high usage is heavily associated with potentially long-term and permanent psychiatric damage. I have been involved in a few cases in which seventeen-year-old lads had each developed a severe psychotic psychiatric illness after a few weeks of heavy cannabis usage. Both had required sectioning and psychiatric unit admission to treat their illnesses, and protect themselves and others from potential danger. Both of these young men still remain ill many years later. Their whole lives are affected and severely impaired, with the inevitable associated massive impact on their families. Newspapers often report 'life-changing injuries' following serious road traffic accidents; perhaps we should also record 'cannabis-triggered life-changing brain injuries' in cases like this.

Like many British towns, ours has a significant illegal drug problem. GPs were often used in the past by addicts to try to get prescription drugs to help them cope with withdrawal or even just to sell at times. GPs were often under a great deal of pressure to try to help addicts, even though they did not want to add to the problem. A variety of government schemes have been attempted in order to try to help addicts reduce or stop their dependency, originally using methadone to help reduce withdrawal symptoms. Evidence had previously shown that areas in which addicts were supported in this way showed massive drops in petty crime, at the very least, let alone the reduction in, less easily measurable, human misery.

Our practice was involved in a number of programmes over the years, often in conjunction with community drug workers. One of the other GPs and I had done extra training to help us with our drug support roles. Along with a number of other practices in our area, we took part in a community drug team (CDT) initiative for several years. This mostly involved a CDT support worker reviewing patients with drug dependence problems regularly in our surgeries, both for our patients and those of other GPs who were not taking part in the scheme. The support workers were uniformly excellent at their job. They reviewed the client's (patient's) current illegal and prescribed drug usage, together with social and family situations. They also arranged urine testing to confirm current drug intakes. The aim being to prescribe methadone or equivalents safely, using a reducing dose to stop or massively curtail illegal drug usage. Patients who were unable to stop were still able to function in society a lot better: holding down jobs and looking after children more safely. My colleague and I would offer general medical and psychiatric support and also had six-monthly face-to-face reviews with each of the CDT clients, alongside the CDT worker. Many of these clients had been using on and off (mostly on) for years, sometimes decades. They were mostly as chaotic as you might imagine.

'How're you doing, Joe?' I asked one at his review. He had previously been a patient of ours but was now with another GP in the area.

'I'm all right, ta, Doctor. Good to see you. You're looking good!' he lied kindly.

'How much are you using?'

'Not much. I'm doin' OK. Just a bit o' weed. And a few Es. Some amphets at weekend. A bit o' coke when I've got the cash. Nowt much.'

'Your urine showed some heroin usage, Joe,' chipped in the CDT worker.

'Oh yeah. You 'ave to, don't yeh? You know how it is?' he answered with a broken-toothed grin.

Not really, but I tried to be empathic and helpful, within limits. Joe's attitude and relaxed use of illegal drugs was and still is widespread, of course. Many drug team reviews were like that one. Nevertheless, overall, the service was excellent and helped patients, and would hopefully also reduce local crime figures.

Stefan's journey was more precipitous. He had briefly attended the CDT clinics, but his drug usage was too chaotic and heavy to allow him to continue in that set-up and he was returned to ordinary GP care: frequently booking emergency appointments, trying to get us to prescribe benzodiazepines or unsupervised methadone (answer: no). He continued to inject heroin and at one time gave himself a stroke as he injected into his neck, accidentally entering his right carotid artery with a whoosh of poorly dissolved drug. He had a reasonable recovery from this severe health warning, with some residual facial weakness only, but his well-being remained imperilled by his lifestyle and he died later that same year, aged thirty-two, following some gang-related violence.

• • •

Another long-term patient, Ronald, was reviewed after Carole, the CDT worker, had given me a quick update. She told me that he had recently been left £20,000 in his gran's will. I dreaded to think how long that would last. Ronald came in and we went through his current drug usage and methadone dose-reduction regime. Towards the end of the consultation, I expressed my condolences about his gran's death. She had also been a patient of ours.

'It's all right. She was ninety-odd, so it's sort of expected, to be fair. Did you know she'd left me £20k?'

'Yes, Carole told me. What're you going to do with that?' I asked, eyebrows raised as I looked across at Carole, who was stood beside Ronald.

'I've just bought a nice sofa for me flat and I'm getting a big wide-screen telly. I'm gettin' an ISA with the rest, so I don't spend it all on drugs.'

Not the answer I'd expected at all. A useful reminder that people can still veer away from the cliched, and expected, path.

Sian

One of the practice regulars was Sian, a young woman in her mid-thirties. She made pre-booked or emergency appointments most weeks, often several. She had four children who she also brought in frequently, usually for straightforward coughs and colds. She seemed to have little support at home, least of all by the fathers of any of her children. Her main problems related to chronic unhappiness, asthma and undiagnosed abdominal pains, although she usually brought an additional long written list of new problems and prescription requests to each consultation.

She had been on six or seven different antidepressant medications and was always keen to try yet another one in case that would give her some breakthrough or boost. My colleagues and I often resisted this and tried to reduce her emotional dependence on medications and doctors. Her usual response was to book an emergency appointment to go back on or try a new medication. Counselling and psychotherapeutic services also struggled to get her to engage. One of my consultations with her had followed a similar pattern of medication requests and new symptoms, ending with what I hoped was a good shared management plan. I handed her a prescription. She remained sitting in her chair and started to rub her podgy belly.

'The baby keeps kicking me and it 'urts,' she said.

I felt a cold sweat appear on my forehead.

'Are you pregnant?' I asked, panicking as I looked at her most recently prescribed medications on the computer screen to see if they were safe in pregnancy. I had no idea she was pregnant again.

'No, the baby keeps kicking me,' she repeated, both helpful and completely unhelpful at the same time.

'Are you pregnant?' I tried again, this time checking whether or not my colleagues had noted this in her records.

'No, I told you. The baby keeps kicking me. When I pick him up!'

'Oh, I see!' I said, finally realising that baby meant her youngest child, a toddler.

She smiled at me, stood up, ready to leave, and said, 'He's a pain. I just wish he'd stop kicking me. Bye.'

She left the room.

Is it me? I wondered as I wrote up the details of the consultation.

I Am a Number, Not a Name

When seeing deaf patients for pre-booked appointments, we often had the opportunity to book sign language interpreters. They were such a boon, especially for helping the patients who had poor lip-reading skills and also those with no speech at all.

On one occasion, one of these skilful interpreters, Joan, was helping with a deaf chap, Robert, who was in his late sixties. Robert could lip-read a certain amount but had little effective speech. He and Joan communicated in British Sign Language (BSL) and Joan and I spoke to each other.

At the end of the consultation, I asked how Joan had come to develop such BSL skills, as she appeared to have no hearing difficulties. She told me that her dad had been born deaf so she had learnt as a child in the home. While talking to me, she continued to sign, of course, so that Robert could follow our conversation. He joined in and asked what school her dad had gone to. It turned out that her dad had attended Manchester Deaf School, as had Robert. Joan continued to speak out loud while they signed so that I could follow their conversation as well. Robert asked Joan what her dad's name was and she replied with what appeared to be a number. He also signed a number back. They both smiled and signed to each other for another minute or so. Robert, in particular, looked quite excited and happy as their conversation went on: nodding and smiling non-stop. It seemed that Joan's dad and Robert had been in the same class at deaf school and she had not found this out till now, even though she had interpreted for Robert many times previously.

I asked why she did not appear to have signed or spoken her dad's name. She told me that all of the children at the deaf school were given a number to use in school, rather than a name. Robert had recognised her dad's number and passed his back to Joan so that she could tell her dad when she next saw him. I said that that it seemed a bit inhuman to use numbers instead of names for small children. She agreed but said that that was just the way it was in 'the old days' and Robert agreed. The school itself had closed years ago in order that deaf children should go to 'normal' schools and integrate better in that way. It was hard to disagree with that sentiment and concept, but Robert and Joan also expressed their belief that the deaf children did enjoy some benefits from the comradeship of mixing with their peers back then. Indeed, Robert was very keen to regain contact with his old school friend, Joan's dad, as soon as they could. Joan told me that they were likely to still use their old school numbers to each other, as her dad had done this previously with other former school friends.

(I understand that there is still a specialised school in the south area of Greater Manchester for deaf students who additionally have severe or complex learning difficulties.)

Bad Hair Day

A patient attended on my duty day on an emergency appointment. She was a smartly dressed middle-aged lady. She sat down and then sat back in the chair.

I started with, 'How can I help you?'

'I need a sick note,' she replied.

'What's wrong?' I asked.

She leant forwards and spoke to me conspiratorially. 'Just put flu.'

'Why, do you think you've got flu?' I asked.

'No, but just put flu.'

'I'm not putting that down if you haven't got it,' I said. 'What is wrong?'

She sat back again, snorted and pointed to her head with both index fingers. I could not work out what any of that meant.

'What?' I tried again.

She repeated the same actions and sounds and then added, 'Look.'

I was none the wiser and told her.

'I'm not going into work till this grows out a bit,' she told me. 'Look at the state of it!'

I was finally the wiser. She had a fairly short and severe haircut.

'You want a sick note for a bad hair day?' I asked with obvious irritation. 'If that was allowed, I'd be able to put in for early retirement.' This being a reference to my nicely progressing baldness.

'You can't blame me for asking,' she said.

I did, indeed, blame her for asking, and for using an emergency appointment to do so.

'I could have just lied,' she continued in her defence, and then, 'I'll just have to use my leave up now.' She got up and left, with a parting shot of, 'Thanks for nothing,' as she slammed the door.

Sick Note

People trust doctors.

People trust doctors with their health and lives, literally.

The government trusts doctors.

The government trusts doctors to look after the health of the population, but also to be a safeguard on sickness claims for work incapacity.

These two roles do not always sit well together and can, in fact, conflict quite heavily with each other in many ways. It is difficult for a GP to completely disagree with a patient's expressed belief about their current level of health or sickness. Much of a person's perceived health relates as much to their pre-existing attitudes to sickness and work as to their actual condition. I have seen many apparently fit and healthy young men who believe that their muscular backache and stiffness should entitle them to permanent disability benefits. Equally, I have seen many severely disabled and ill patients who want to work and feel that their human rights are being compromised by not being allowed to. Obviously, these are two extremes, but we all recognise this picture.

Starting with sick notes: GPs used to be expected to provide these from the third day of a person's declared sickness. It was, thankfully, realised that having all of these patients getting (or trying to get) an appointment with their GP for a sick note for a short illness was unnecessary, unless actual medical advice or help was needed as well. The period of self-certification was extended to a week in order to help ease this pressure on General Practice, but a note is then required if the illness or sickness continues beyond that. I note that a doctor's sick note (now known as a 'fit note', in part as encouragement of an attitude of expected return to work rather than chronic sickness) is then required. This can apparently now also be provided by an 'Allied Health Professional' instead. This secondary list includes osteopaths, chiropractors, herbalists, acupuncturists and Christian Scientists (yes, really: see the government website). This list was also further extended in 2022 to include, among others, pharmacists, nurses and physiotherapists.

If a person remains unwell or unfit, the GP (or Christian Scientist!) may issue ongoing fit notes for up to six months in total. From that time on, the DSS will generally take over the assessment and issuing of further notes. This change is meant to have benefits of having an independent assessment of the claimant's health, perhaps absolving the GP from being overgenerous to the patient who they know and may feel forced to help against their best judgement. It was also meant to reduce the need for unnecessary GP appointments if there was no other reason for booking this. All very well so far, you might think. The problems often begin when a patient is in conflict with the result of their assessment, particularly when they are declared fit but don't agree. At that point, if they wish to appeal, they are expected to see their GP, who is, of course, then expected to support them, often by offering an exaggerated interpretation of the sickness and its effects on the person. Failure to help, or try to help, is not looked upon kindly by the patient, who you will continue to see for many years. And their family, as well.

GPs are, naturally, used to saying no to patients who request drugs or referrals that they can't have and will still refuse to lie for such an appeal. However, the conflict and awkwardness will remain. This can present ongoing problems with the future GP–patient relationship or the more worrying tendency to try to bend the truth a little to help the patient. In addition, GPs are also (usually high-rate) taxpayers and feel a responsibility for not wasting government (our) money, too.

This potential conflict also continues within other roles that GPs carry with regard to other benefit applications and appeals. The elephant in the room is the nature of many benefits and the spurious linkage to health. Then there is the precipitous benefits trap itself, within which many people find themselves, where any attempt to escape often leads to a drop in income, at least for a while. Often, the only solution for people caught in this trap is to declare themselves as even sicker or more disabled. All of this has led to a massive increase, in the last twenty years, in the number of people who are registered as disabled in the UK. It is hard to believe that there could have been a real increase in illness and disability in a country such as this, with free healthcare and ever safer conditions in the workplace.

I don't think that 'The System' itself necessarily always helps people to escape even when they are feeling better. Many stop wanting to and make their own plans to never consider working again.

Many patients – even those who are young – say, when asked, about jobs, 'I don't work.' Often this relates to their stated belief that their mental health will not allow them to ever work, as if they will never feel any better. This is often stated by patients with no evidence or symptoms related to significant disease, such as bipolar disease, schizophrenia, psychotic depression, obsessive-compulsive disorder (OCD), severe anxiety, severe depression, eating disorders or postnatal depression.

I had a consultation with a woman in her twenties called Leanne, who had booked an appointment to review her anti-depressant medications. She told me that she still felt low and wondered if she might try a different drug: this would be her seventh different antidepressant, but this new wonder drug had been recommended to her by a friend. I discussed this with her, particularly the very small chance that this drug would be dramatically better than the previous six. I wondered if she might want to consider another referral to the community mental health team. She remained keen to try the other medication and not keen to pursue any other referral.

Item two on her agenda was for me to help support her appeal against a potential benefit drop. I understood this related to a change from Disability Living Allowance (DLA) to Personal Independence Payment (PIP). She was keen that I should write a letter, specifically stressing that her mental health condition was never going to improve.

It is very difficult to reconcile those two intentions and requirements in a single consultation. She wanted to feel better but at the same time wanted written confirmation from me that she never would. Leanne may well have been playing the system to her benefit (literally), but had also found herself stuck within the benefit black hole. She would either need to make big changes to her expectations or get a fairly decent job to escape the moderately comfortable income she was currently receiving. Neither of these seemed likely.

Guilt

Sharon, a former nurse in her mid-fifties, came to see Bernadette, who was the practice registrar at that time. Sharon
explained that she had a lump in her breast, but initially did not
want to talk much more about how long she had known about
it. She requested that she wanted it to be examined first. Bernadette examined her and was a bit shocked to find a very large
and obvious hard tumour in Sharon's right breast. This felt like a
definite and well-established cancer. Bernadette explained this
to Sharon and told her that she would complete an urgent referral to the local breast clinic for proper diagnosis and treatment.
She would be seen within two weeks. She then asked if Sharon
had any idea about the nature of this lump and wondered how
long she had known about it. Sharon then told her the story
behind the lump.

She said that she also thought it was probably cancer and had
actually first noticed it over three years ago, but did not want to
see a doctor about it at that time. Her reason for this was that
her daughter was just about to start at university at that time and
she did not want to distract from or upset her time at university. During her work as a nurse, she had seen the impact that
a cancer diagnosis and treatment had on the patient and their
families and wanted to prevent any such effects on her daughter's
education and career. Her daughter had now got her degree and
had recently started in a good job. Sharon felt that she could now
come forward for help without potentially impacting her daughter's future prospects too much.

Bernadette was shocked and upset at this worrying and
potentially fatal sacrifice, and found it very hard not to shout out

with frustration or any direct criticism, as she was keen to engage Sharon on her future treatment plan.

Sharon was diagnosed with a high-grade cancer and underwent surgery and radiotherapy. It is too soon to know whether or not her delay in seeking treatment has led to it being ineffective. I wonder how her poor daughter has reacted to her mum's illness, and I wonder if she has ever been told of the delay in seeking treatment and the reasons for this. There are often complex feelings of guilt and uselessness already when a loved one becomes ill, but these would likely be even harder to bear in this case.

Bernadette is a kind and thoughtful person and doctor, and was also greatly affected and upset by this lady's story. She talked to me about the impact that the case had on her feelings and also put it in writing in her training portfolio. We were able to discuss ways in which doctors can try to cope with the sort of emotions generated by some of the stresses of General Practice. Some emotional detachment from patients' pain and suffering is essential in order to work as a doctor, otherwise the job would be nigh-on impossible. Nevertheless, some cases really hit home, often when the patient is a similar age to yourself or to a family member.

Ghosts

One of the joys and privileges of General Practice is being able to visit patients in their homes. Many of the most precious of consultations take place on these visits; the most severely ill patients are often seen there, especially for end-of-life care. We also used to do early postnatal home visits to check up on new mums and babies.

Visiting can also, of course, be one of the greatest nuisances, as visit requests often come in at the most awkward moments, such as when you are just starting a three- to four-hour evening surgery. Especially if the visit could and should have been requested a bit earlier.

Our catchment area was around six miles across, which is quite large for an urban practice, but I got to know most of it fairly well over my thirty-odd years working there. Driving around, it is hard not to feel some responsibility for the patients that you see, out and about and shopping. I often wondered if that is how clergymen and women feel about their flocks. Every street also contains memories of patients seen at home there, often those with chronic and terminal illnesses. I remember many of these housebound folk, hidden and suffering behind normal-looking front doors. Some bed-bound, others on home oxygen therapy, lots needing frequent carer visits or round-the-clock care, often done by struggling relatives, who carry such a heavy and unseen burden.

Without trying to sound too dramatic, I also feel an aware-ness of all the patients who have passed away, like ghosts, hover-ing just out of sight in every street. This is one of the reasons that I did not feel comfortable living within the practice boundary.

Of course, a similar pattern of illnesses and death will cover all but the newest roads across the country, including mine, but I prefer not to know. I am very happy for my neighbours to keep their anonymity and privacy as much as I keep mine.

Another more pleasant thing I associated with visiting was the chance to listen to the car radio, in my case usually tuned to Radio 2. This was frequently a reminder of life outside our practice boundary, of well people getting on with their normal lives, and often more glamorous activities than many of my patients were motivated or able to do.

Occasionally, however, the frequent references to 'prosecco o'clock' and posh glamping weekends in yurts could get a bit irritating.

The best thing on Radio 2, though, by far, was Ken Bruce's *PopMaster* quiz. An absolute joy to hear this at 10.30 a.m. on weekdays, so I would often park up for ten minutes to listen to this whenever I was able before getting on with the rest of my home visits. I still try to catch the programme and quiz now, despite Ken jumping ship and taking *PopMaster* with him to another broadcaster, as well as the occasional TV version, too.

Behind the Door

I did a visit to the home of one of our patients. She and her children always attended the surgery immaculately turned out, wearing the latest designer gear. I called to see one of her children. The house looked reasonable from outside, particularly the smart new Audi parked on the drive. Inside was a total mess, including piles of dog muck liberally spread throughout the ground floor, with everybody just stepping around the piles as if they were patterns on the lino. Several teenagers were sitting and watching the massive TV, tutting while I walked in front of it, navigating the poo minefield. I saw and examined their poorly sibling upstairs before telling Mum about the health hazard of the dog waste. She shrugged and blamed the teenagers, telling me she was more worried about the state of her children's health rather than the house, as I should also be; perhaps missing the point.

Several other properties were a source of shock, often due to the amount of hoarding, the most severe often being seen in Diogenes syndrome, also known as senile squalor syndrome, which is often observed in patients with dementia or other frontal-lobe brain diseases. In many cases, this leads to storage of rubbish and, basically, keeping everything that most of us would normally throw out. The smell was usually overwhelming, especially in the face of the apparent lack of awareness by the patient, who often otherwise appeared to have no problems if they were seen outside their home.

Other severe cases of hoarding I've seen have been in homes of well-educated people with obsessional traits but no formally diagnosed illness. In one extreme example, I visited the home of a patient and her two middle-aged sons who had never married nor left home. The mum had early dementia but both sons were working in fairly good jobs, although both seemed to lack normal social skills and awareness. When first visiting, I was shown through the house, basically via a very narrow corridor between newspapers, magazines and books piled to the ceiling, eight feet high. This corridor started at the front door and continued through the hall, up the stairs and across the landing into her bedroom. All of the windows were obscured by the piles of paper. Most of the rooms appeared to be set out the same way, with just a two-foot-wide pathway leading to chairs, sinks and toilets.

When confronting the sons with the dangers of this level of hoarding, both shrugged their shoulders and said they would sort it out when they got the time. One of them was particularly obsessed with trains and all of his magazines and books related to this topic, and the other with some aspect of local history, which I have forgotten. Neither showed any real desire or willingness to confront the issue. Their mum required help and care from the district nurses as well as ourselves for a while before she went into a care home. I don't think any of my colleagues have visited the family home since, but I doubt that either son has voluntarily cleared any of their collections. They may even have celebrated having a few more square feet of storage available in their mum's bedroom.

Alternative

We all look for improvements in health and well-being, even if we have exhausted the apparent resources of our healthcare providers to enhance our lot.

Previously, doctors would surreptitiously prescribe placebo drugs in order to effect psychological improvements in patients' symptoms, or sometimes medications of small or dubious benefit given in a similar fashion. It was hoped that they might help a bit, but at least each method was unlikely to be harmful. This kind of underhand non-treatment is now frowned upon as being dishonest and patronising, with honesty being rightfully encouraged. Maybe this is a slight shame, as the placebo effect does work a little and it also demonstrated to the patient that you were appearing to take them seriously and trying to help.

Understandably, patients look for other ways to manage their symptoms if doctors do not appear to have any more to offer.

Complementary therapies can be a great help in easing symptoms and giving you a lift, of course. Who doesn't enjoy being a bit pampered and comforted by spa and massage treatments, for example? Many of these treatments are feel-good therapies that promote a lift in mental health symptoms, and are often used in tandem with medical treatments; being offered in hospice care, for instance. The practitioners of many of these treatments can also suggest likely benefits well beyond any actual physical improvements, thus embracing the placebo effect in a way that medical doctors no longer can.

Alternative therapies vary greatly and can include herbal remedies, reflexology and homeopathy, for instance. Many of the treatments appear of no scientific benefit whatsoever, but you might argue that they are unlikely to harm as they are 'natural'. Lots of poisons are natural and so that particular argument does not hold up very well. I have also seen two patients who have developed severe liver damage after years of taking a harmful herbal medication. Remembering that if any ingested treatment may be helpful, then it will of course have the potential to cause side effects, allergies or other physical harm. Another harm can be raising false hope in people, or maybe just losing their money on a waste of time and effort. Sometimes even *our* money, as the NHS has itself spent plenty of money on homeopathy: a bizarre, disproven belief system bordering on a religion.

Patients frequently came to see me to ask what the best alternative medicine was for their condition.

Patient, Gemma, suffering from irritable bowel syndrome (IBS) – 'I didn't like those tablets that consultant, Dr Bromley, gave me and the ones you gave me were worse.'

Me – 'Sorry to hear that. What was the problem with the new one?'

Gemma – 'They gave me a dry mouth.'

Me – 'OK, that is fairly common with that type of tablet. There are other different medications that we can look at if you would like?'

Gemma – 'Well, I was hoping for some help with alternative medicine.'

Me – 'Well, that's not really my field.'

Gemma – 'Well, you're here to help me with whatever I ask.'

Me – 'Not necessarily, and not with alternative medicines.'

Gemma – 'Why not?'

Me – 'Because it's alternative to me. There's a clue in the title.'

Gemma – 'Well, I don't expect you to prescribe it for me; I'll buy it.'

Me – 'As I said, it's alternative to the scientific methods that I have been taught in and studied. All the meds that we prescribe have been tested at different doses in different people, and their side effects and interactions with other drugs have been tested. Any unexpected effects are recorded and reported. Alternative medicines haven't been.'

Gemma – 'Well, they're all just plants, so they can't do any harm.'

Me – 'That's not true. Some plants are poisonous. I'm not against the use of treatments derived from plants, as many of the meds we use have come from nature. It's just that they have been refined and purified into doses that we know about.'

Gemma – 'So you won't help me?'

Me – 'If you tell me what you plan to take, I can see if there is any information on its safety or its interactions with your diabetic meds, for instance.'

Gemma – 'But you won't tell me what to buy?'

Me – 'No, but I am happy to look at other licenced treatments for you.'

A much more commonly used and requested 'alternative treatment' request was for cannabis, for whatever disease the patient already had and that they were already usually smoking. Cannabis products were only actually licensed for a very narrow list of conditions and prescribing was limited to a very few specially licensed doctors only. I suggested to several patients that in years to come, some refined cannabis products may become available and may be prescribable as a proper or real drug, like all the other meds in the BNF. Most of the patients requesting it then stated that they wouldn't want it then, as it would no longer be alternative enough for them.

Memories

Patients with dementia, and also other chronic mental health problems, are encouraged to have an annual practice review of their physical health. The reviews are most commonly done by nurses, although in some practices the GPs also do them.

I was undertaking one of these reviews with a patient in her nineties, Annie. She had dementia with very severe recent memory loss and had been brought in by a professional carer. While doing the review, it was quite evident just how severe Annie's memory loss was: she did not know who the carer was, nor who I was, nor why she was here. I had known her for over twenty years.

I asked the carer whether Annie seemed any clearer at other times when she was at home or in other environments. She told me that Annie attended a day care centre and that there were old school photographs on the walls in many of the rooms there. One of the school group photographs was of Annie's primary school. Annie recognised herself in the photograph and was able to name every one of the other eleven girls. The carer now had a copy of this photo on her phone and showed it to me and then to Annie, who once more recognised and named all the girls, including herself. Remarkably, three of the other girls on the picture also now had dementia and attended the same day care centre. They had come full circle and were back together again towards the end of their lives. Maybe I should have been able to find some reassurance or comfort in this fact, but it made me feel incredibly sad.

It still does.

I think it struck a nerve in me because the full potential cycle of their lives, perhaps all of our lives, was on such evident display in this group of friends – dependent childhood through independent adulthood and back to the childlike state of needing support and care again. It also showed that quite a high ratio of that class had developed dementia – one in three at that particular time, that we were aware of. Others in the group may have moved away or developed a similar condition earlier or later than this particular group.

Doctors' Letters

Patients ask GPs to write letters for them for all kinds of reasons: many of these are formal and necessary; others are informal but useful; some are just plain bizarre. Sometimes officials request unnecessary GP letters from patients as an avoidance or delaying tactic, knowing that they will be refused or, God forbid, charged for.

Many patients have to approach GPs in order to access different levels of benefits and support, so it is not my intention to criticise them for this. I realise that the whole system is flawed and over-medicalised and that even token contact with the health service is seen as giving some enhanced credibility to claims. All those who work in this system are aware of inherent flaws, as are many of the patients. The NHS has enough to do in managing current illnesses and also trying to prevent future disease, but a good proportion of patients are competing with benefit claimants for appointments to access the NHS because of the bureaucratic demands of the UK social security arrangements.

I was once asked for a note to excuse a woman's son from having to wear goggles at school swimming lessons, in order to stop the other children from 'twanging' them at him. I declined and suggested that she continue to try to sort this out with the teachers if it was a big worry.

On another occasion, I was asked for a letter by a mum, so that her eleven-year-old son could attend the secondary school of his choice. This placement had been refused by the local authority as he lived well outside the catchment area. Mum told me he was distraught, although her chubby son sat, smiling and seemingly oblivious, in the chair between us. I replied that I didn't feel this was a medical matter. She then told me that he would kill himself if he was not given his school choice. He appeared distracted and not very interested.

'Tell him,' she said to him. 'Tell him what you're going to do if you can't go to that school.'

'Now?' he muttered.

'Yes,' she replied. 'Go on.'

'Yeah, I think I might kill myself.'

I did not believe, of course, that this boy was as bothered about this school as his mum was and felt that this presentation was a complete set-up by the mum. I was also upset that she was schooling her son in using emotional blackmail to get what he, or in this case, she, wanted. I refused to get involved in this charade and had serious concerns about the emotional impact of this behavioural manipulation.

I asked him and the mum a few questions to try to establish whether he appeared to have any genuine underlying emotional or psychological issues. Everything appeared fine. I suggested referring him to our local children's mental health unit because of the worrying statement he had made, although presumably he had been schooled in this.

'Oh, I don't think he'll actually do anything. He's just upset. If you'll just do us that letter, I'm sure he'll be all right,' said the mum. 'And I'll pay you for it.'

No, and no thanks.

Mum was no happier at me saying no to her than she had been about the local education authority's response. She was angry and shocked at my refusal to help her, and threatened to see one of my colleagues. I suggested that she was entitled to do that if she wanted but I doubted that the outcome would be any different. I also told her that I would still be making a referral for her son in view of his statement and her allegation.

I checked up a few weeks later and she had not booked another GP appointment for herself or her son, and had cancelled the referral I'd made.

I have been asked for letters on many occasions by patients who would prefer not to attend court hearings, as they feel stressed or depressed or anxious at the thought of potential imprisonment. One of my colleagues, Norman, did such a letter under pressure from one of his patients. He was summoned to attend court, in place of the accused, by an angry judge. Norman, and the rest of us, found it much easier to refuse such requests thereafter.

Another disturbing but frequent source of letter requests was from asylum seekers, particularly from men of Iraqi and Iranian extraction. We had a series of these patients over a few years: all of them had been refused asylum and all of them followed the same subsequent pattern of presenting illness. They presented with symptoms of severe depression following asylum refusal and each repeatedly threatened suicide and attempted overdoses the nearer we got to their appeal or proposed repatriation date. After attending A&E, a further GP appointment was usually gained where they might request a letter to take to their appeal lawyers to confirm that they were suicidal and would kill themselves if their appeal was refused, or repatriation attempts continued. It is hard not to have sympathy for people in this position, either being made so ill by their circumstances or having to exaggerate their responses in order to try to manipulate the system.

As GPs we also felt very much caught up in the middle of a situation beyond our control. A practice colleague was told by one of these patients that he had been given a list of advice from his asylum counsellor. The list included a stepwise approach, initially presenting at the GP's surgery with escalating symptoms of depression and suicidal intention, culminating in actual 'mild' overdose attempts and repeated presentations at A&E.

We had already suspected some collusion between the men from their remarkably similar presenting patterns of illness and attendance, but my colleague was shocked to hear that they were being so cold-bloodedly coached to block the legal process. It was quite difficult to challenge each patient at their time of presentation, as depression may be an understandable and almost normal response to the threat of repatriation to a potentially dangerous country.

Any letters written by myself or colleagues were to confirm only the known events and made no predictions about potential future behaviour of the patients. I understand that all the patients referred to here did win the right stay in the UK, even if it was just temporary and in order to continue their ongoing asylum appeals.

One of our patients had applied to join the RAF but had been rejected on the grounds of his previous psychiatric illness; he had a history of depression and several overdose attempts and subsequent hospital admissions. He wrote to me at the surgery, asking for me to write a letter suggesting that the RAF should ignore his medical history on the grounds that he had not really been very depressed, and had not really tried hard to kill himself in the past, and that his behaviour was only a response to a bad relationship he'd been in at that time. He stated that he would promise never to attempt an overdose or suicide again.

Many branches of the government are used to bending over to try to accommodate a person's previous health problems. The RAF is, of course, not one of these organisations, nor would most people expect it to be. If somebody does not want to take responsibility for their own actions then, it is fair to say, that you may not want to trust them to fly a £100 million plane loaded with missiles and bombs.

I wrote back to the patient, sympathetically, to inform that him I could not override their health records and nor would the

RAF accept my word that he would never be depressed again in the future. I discussed the letters with my colleague, Masud, and he produced a slightly more inappropriate and amusing response letter of his own – with no intention to post, thankfully:

Dear Mr X,

We have received your recent email advising that the RAF have rejected your application as 'medically unfit' due to your history of multiple self-harm/suicidal intents in the past three years. I appreciate that you were going through a stressful time in your life, which has now resolved, and that you no longer intend to self-harm, as stipulated in your letter. This, unfortunately, will still not be acceptable to join the RAF as they have very stringent mental health requirements for what can be a stressful job.

However, all is not lost.

I have been making some enquiries and if you still wish to pursue a career in flying, then the Japanese Air Force will gladly accept you within one of their elite units. Please let me know how you would like to proceed and I can do a letter addressed to their Kamikaze Training Branch.

Yours (In)Sincerely,

Dr Z

War Wound

Like most urban or inner city areas, we have a broad ethnic and cultural mix of patients, with many born overseas. When I first started, the greatest numbers of these were from the Indian subcontinent, but with increasing numbers from Eastern and Central Europe over time. The largest single influx we had at any one time was when a large group of refugees from the Balkans conflict were moved into a nearby tower block. We were happy to accept the request for all of these patients to join our practice list. At that time, there was obviously a great deal of sympathy and goodwill towards them because of the horrendous suffering that they had been through; there were many similarities to the current Ukraine conflict, although the Balkan Wars had already ended when the refugees arrived in the UK. We expected an initial rush for appointments to sort out these patients' long-neglected health problems and made extra slots available. We also had access to translators, as most of these new patients had very little English when they first arrived.

Tarik was one of the first of these patients who I saw, together with the translator, Hana. Tarik was a sturdy and serious-looking chap in his early forties. He wore a heavy black leather jacket on this hot summer's day.

I welcomed him, via the translator, and he thanked me back. I gained the impression that these two did not really get on well, as they seemed to be snarling at each other a little and I was not sure how accurately the translator was communicating between us. It reminded me of some of the translators in Botswana when I was a student. Some of them had appeared to be inserting their own agendas or trying to block any in-depth consultations. Back in Tarik's session, and we eventually seemed to get to the main point of today's consultation. Tarik extended his left hand to me and I could see that it was badly scarred. I examined it more closely and realised that he was unable to fully extend his fingers, having a fixed flexion deformity from the injury and scarring. I asked how he had injured his hand, expecting a story of bullets or shrapnel from some fighting in the conflict he had escaped. It took Hana some time to convey the reality to me, particularly as Tarik appeared to be re-enacting a massive explosion of sorts, but the injury seemed to have been caused by a sewing machine. Presumably a large factory machine rather than a small domestic one, but nevertheless not quite what I'd expected, especially from his expansive mime.

I referred him to a hand surgeon who, over time and together with a plastic surgeon, was able to effect some improvement in Tarik's hand function. I also realised that the apparent disquiet between Tarik and Hana seemed to be repeated in most other consultations with this group and their translators. I now realise that this was just evidence of a cultural difference between how they interact with each other, compared to how British people tend to. A difference that I have seen repeated many times since visiting parts of Eastern Europe, characterised by most people looking unhappy and not smiling very much, at least in public.

The Myth of Consent

Throughout medical training, practitioners are encouraged to explain options to patients properly and to gain appropriate consent from them. This is meant to be 'informed' consent, meaning that a full explanation of the likely pathway of an illness and on the different available treatments has first been given. All of this is meant to be explained in an appropriate and understandable way to any given patient or family, depending on their culture and educational levels of understanding. This is far different from the old-style approach of a doctor telling the patient what the doctor plans to do and seeking a vague acceptance or agreement by the patient, followed by thrusting a form in front of them and saying, 'Sign here.'

I often received hospital clinic or discharge letters stating that the doctor had 'consented' the patient to a given procedure, as if the consent was done *to* the patient rather than *by* them. The phrase may have been used as a kind of shorthand to explain a more complicated process, but words matter and may reflect or influence the attitudes of other doctors.

This led me to think more generally about the use and, perhaps, misuse of informed consent in medical practice.

Thinking, firstly, of working in surgical specialities. When surgeons advise on acute problems, such as appendicitis, which appear to merit surgery as perhaps the only credible treatment, surgeons tend not to offer a wide range of alternative management plans. They suggest surgery *only*, and expect automatic consent despite the potential risks that should have been explained. So much is their consent assumed that if the patient refuses surgery, they are not even offered an alternative treatment. In fact, patients may even be asked to sign a different form altogether – one that suggests they refuse to take the medical advice that has been offered.

On other occasions, it seems that informed consent for planned surgery is weaponised in such a way as to convince willing participants to think again, especially the elderly and ill. It may well, of course, be prudent and sensible to dissuade the patient, particularly if the patient is actually very frail or has underlying medical problems that skew the risk–benefit ratio markedly towards risk. I just think that the consent form or procedure itself is not best used as the main communication tool. Patients have often told me that they were given a list of rare possible complications of surgery, presented as being very likely or inevitable.

Moving away from surgical procedures, which, as outlined here, generally require written consent, how many *non-surgical* management plans involve proper consent for procedures or prescriptions? Of course, doctors should develop shared management plans with the patient – indeed, this is a cornerstone of sensible medical practice. This is certainly taught, encouraged and measured throughout the student and postgraduate medical training process. Do doctors, though, always really explain, fully, the consequences and importance of undertaking blood tests and scans?

The formal consent previously required for HIV testing appears to have been downgraded somewhat, perhaps in recognition of access to better drugs and treatments, making the disease much less threatening than it was previously perceived to be. However, many other pathology tests and imaging procedures regularly reveal often unexpected but life-threatening diseases, and formal consent is rarely sought for these investigations.

When it comes to prescribing medications, do doctors fully explore several alternatives and request written consent for the drugs that they prescribe, and that may have serious future impact upon patients' lives and well-being? Should they ask for written consent to prescribe, or even more, not to prescribe? Is consent presumed by patients accepting a script, or by having it dispensed, or upon taking the drug after having first read the Patient Information Leaflet?

What about full consent with regard to the range of possible shared management plans?

How many alternative plans should actually be offered? Maybe two, with a token unlikely bonus one thrown in? Should doctors be neutral in their presentation of alternative plans or should they pretend to be, while heavily encouraging patients towards their preference?

Doctors are only human, for now at least,* and it has been suggested being completely non-directive may be non-helpful! It is no wonder that many patients seek more directive help elsewhere with alternative practitioners, who have no worries about what treatments they have absolute faith in, however misguided.

When I, myself, have been discussing different possible treatments for my own medical care, I have sometimes asked the clinician, 'What would you do?' Not an easy question to answer while trying to be neutral, but a very helpful answer for the patient to hear.

The point of this brief chapter is not just to judge or criticise. Doctors and patients are all caught up in this. I just believe that doctors are kidding themselves if they feel that we are completely neutral in the process of offering treatments and receiving consent. Also, the range of management options that

---

* Although artificial intelligence (AI) is apparently primed to take up an increasingly large role in the future provision of medical care.

they do not currently gain written consent for may have just as major an impact on future health as those that they currently, routinely, do.

Things People Say ...

During a consultation with a patient called Ruth, who had booked her appointment hoping for a steroid injection into her knee, I asked, 'Which knee is it?'

Ruth pointed to her right knee. 'This is the worse one, by far ...'

After a short pause, she then pointed to her left knee and said, 'And this one's just as bad.'

Many patients, on being asked about the current problem – 'I don't know where to start.'

Me, after hearing this a few hundred times – 'Near the end would be good.'

In a similar, perhaps slightly cynical, vein.

Many patients – 'Ooh, I could write a book.'

Me, to patients – 'Ooh, you should. That would be interesting.'

Me, to self – 'I wish you would, then I could decide if I wanted to read it, as opposed to being forced to listen.'

Me, to many patients, as directed by a lifetime of training and good, caring and sharing, General Practice – 'What do you think the problem is?'

Many patients – 'You tell me. You're the doctor.' Often accompanied by a scrunched-up face and glance to their partner, invariably present in the room and chuckling along.

Me, to patient and inevitable sidekick – 'Well, I'm not a vet, so you are allowed to give an opinion.'

Me, to self – 'Although it's likely to be ridiculous.'

Patient in her thirties, offended at being reported to social services by a neighbour – 'I only left the kids to get a ten bag o' weed.'

She continued, 'I wish I had cancer: I'm that fed up!'

Me, wondering how long I can even attempt or pretend to show any more empathy or interest – 'That is a ridiculous and offensive thing to say.'

She, defensively – 'Well, I'd get more attention if I did.'

Me – 'Do you really want that kind of attention? I see people every day whose lives and families are wrecked by cancer.'

She – 'Anything'd be good. It's not fair.'

And so it went on.

Patient in her mid-eighties: lovely lady, Ingrid, who was born in Austria and still had a strong accent despite living in the UK since the 1940s. She came in for a review appointment early one January.

Ingrid – 'Did you have a good Christmas, Doctor?'

Me – 'Yes, thanks. It was busy here until Christmas Eve, but it was lovely to have Christmas and Boxing Day off.'

Ingrid – 'Did you see your family?'

Me – 'Yes, we had most of them over for Christmas dinner and saw the rest on Boxing Day. What about you?'

Ingrid – 'Well, you know my daughter; she is very kind. We were at her family's house all day over the holidays and then they took us home at night, full of drink and food. She bought me a lovely fudge bar.'

I was a little surprised at this, as her daughter and son-in-law ran several very successful businesses in the area. They had a lovely house with a swimming pool and they both drove top-end cars.

Me – 'A fudge bar?'

Ingrid – 'Yes. Have you tried one?'

Me – 'Err. Yes, but they are a bit sweet for me.'

It was her turn to look a bit confused.

She said – 'Well, they bought me a fancy one. My feet have never felt so good.'

Me – 'A fudge bar?'

Ingrid – 'Yes, you put your feet in and fill it with water. It massages your feet all over. It is lovely.'

Me – 'Oh, a foot spa!'

Ingrid – 'Yes, a fudge bar. You should buy your mother one.'

'That's a good idea. I might,' I said while musing about which of the two she might prefer.

Overweight chap in his thirties, attending in the hope of getting a prescription for Orlistat, a drug that decreases fat absorption from the diet and can help weight loss. There were quite specific criteria around the prescribing of this drug, based on a person's body mass index (BMI): a weight to height ratio.

Me – 'You are overweight, as you know, but not enough to allow me to prescribe Orlistat.'

Him – 'Well, I'll put a few stone on, then, so you'll have to give it me.'

Me – 'So you're saying that you will put weight on so that you can have tablets to help get your weight back to your current weight?'

Him – 'Absolutely. It's my right. Junkies get everything they want from the NHS. For free!'

'Your guess is as good as mine, Doc,' said Robin, a confident cockney chap in his forties, about his abdominal pain.

I was a little taken aback, as I had been trying to explain the diagnosis and my planned confirmatory investigations to him.

I replied sniffily, 'I don't think so.'

'Don't put yourself down, Doc; I'm sure you'll get there in the end. As I said, your guess is as good as mine.'

I had rather presumed that my training and experience had offered me some skill in proffering a more accurate 'guess' than

Robin's and told him so. He remained unmoved and continued to repeat the annoying phrase, so I gave up and just arranged the scan, which later confirmed my guess (gallstones).

Old Friends

The NHS is a marvellous institution, of course: much celebrated and adored; being heavily featured as a thing of great pride even during the London Olympics Opening Ceremony.

I am proud to have worked within it for all of my adult life, but I am not immune to its faults and nor do I believe that my opinion on it is any more important than anybody else's. We all have an emotional investment in it, like a family member. Like a family member, it can also be a source of great irritation, frustration and shame. Also like an errant family member, we feel we have the right to criticise it but don't necessarily enjoy others from outside doing the same.

The best aspect of our system, of course, is that it's free at the point of delivery, paid for by us all from general taxation, at intentionally higher rates from the wealthier citizens. This seems like a good thing to most of us in the UK, but is viewed as a thing of amazement and disgust to many in the USA, for instance.

The US healthcare system is often lauded as exemplary, especially for those who have private insurance rather than the twenty-eight million who don't. But even being fully insured there often leads to over-investigation and over-treatment, which can have its own risks. People often get the care they request, rather than that which is actually needed for their health. It also costs an awful lot more than the NHS, per head, and appears even more inefficient. US-based healthcare providers may beg to differ, of course, and even appear keen to take over the most straightforward bits of NHS care – at great potential profit, naturally.

The downside of our universally free care is that many of us take it so completely for granted that it's sometimes not fully appreciated and we all look for the faults, which are mostly caused by years of overall underfunding. Attempts to overcome or cover for this underfunding have, from different governing political parties, been to try to make the NHS appear more efficient and consumer-led, but as the actual patient is not the payer, it is hard to make this leap in the real world.

Current debate about funding the NHS often features suggestions that we should consider switching to an insurance-based system. This would be a massive financial shock for most people, even to members of private health schemes, as their subscription charges do not currently provide expensive emergency cover, nor many of the more complex things, which the NHS looks after. On the opposite side, it would also appear to be a regression in current income tax rules, as you would expect the NHS element to be removed from this, leaving lower earners to be required to pay relatively more overall. Can you imagine the complaints about higher taxpayers being treated so favourably to the detriment of poorer people?

Frequent and constant top-down reorganisation also has a negative impact on NHS staff morale and functioning, with many feeling a loss of autonomy and control in their workplace. Sometimes changes that are helpful for one part of clinical practice are extended well beyond their usefulness.

A relatively trivial example is banning wearing ties, wrist-watches and full-length sleeves for clinical staff on hospital wards. Well-intentioned, in order to prevent cross infection, and hopefully this has helped hospitals in that regard. The policy was then brought into General Practice, as part of our infection-control procedures, even being policed by the Care Quality Commission (CQC). The problem with this directive is that the average GP consultation room is very different from the average hospital ward or clinic, with a vastly lower chance of any open wounds being cross-contaminated there. Many GPs will not see an open wound from one month to the next and those who undertake minor surgery or other clinical procedures will then adjust their clothing and remove ties and watches, and also add appropriate PPE when required. The last time I checked, there was very insubstantial evidence of any proven benefit of any kind for these changes being imposed on us, too. As I say, a fairly trivial example but an unnecessary and irritating rule change to add to the frequent load of newly imposed rules. In fairness, I think that most younger male GPs no longer even own ties anyway and they rarely wear watches either, even away from work, so perhaps my irritation is more a sign of my age.

The worst thing about the underfunded and overstretched service is that most parts of it are working at maximum capacity most of the time, so that it takes little extra strain to overwhelm the service and create waiting lists. God forbid that any healthcare staff may have a quiet day, say in A&E, and therefore have enough staff capacity to be able to cope when things get busy. Long waits to see GPs and long waits to access any secondary care investigations or treatments also have immense consequences for all of us, with prolongation of human misery and potentially worse outcomes.

Everybody working in the NHS is aware of, and conscious of, common delays and spend a lot of time apologising to patients as a consequence. Patients become used to this state of affairs as the norm and feel free to complain, sometimes even when things are going well.

For example, a middle-aged patient called Bruce.

'Good morning,' I said.

'Morning,' he replied.

'How can I help?'

'I've got a list,' he replied. 'I only had one problem when I booked the appointment, but you know what it's like getting in here. It takes weeks. It's shocking. The NHS is going to pot.'

I looked at his booking details on my computer and spoke again. 'It says here that you booked this appointment yesterday afternoon.'

Bruce's cheeks reddened, but he gave no apology for lying to me. 'Well, it normally takes ages so you have to be ready for that. I'll start with the first three main problems ...'

• • •

'The last time I saw you, you had your finger stuck up my bottom.'

I was standing outside the crematorium, having attended the funeral of a former colleague. Very sad, as you would expect, especially as my colleague had passed away only a few years after retirement. Many other former colleagues were there, and most of an age at which they may have been wondering who might be the next to go. Much of the chatting was about their and their spouses' health problems.

The husband of one of our former administration staff walked briskly across the courtyard towards me. I recognised him as a former patient, too. He shouted out, loudly: 'Hi, Martin. The last time I saw you, you had your finger stuck up my bottom.'

I smiled. I could do little else. I remembered seeing and referring him urgently with a very likely rectal cancer.

'I just wanted to thank you,' he added kindly, and more quietly, and then told us about some of the treatments he had gone through in the years since I last saw him. He was also rightfully pleased to share the news that he had been given the all clear. He was very positive and upbeat and made light of the ongoing downsides of his condition. It was good to hear some relatively good news on that bleak day.

I also got the chance to speak to a few of my current and retired GP colleagues. I reminded one of them, Norman, about his role in an explosion at this very crematorium. Explosions in crematorium ovens are a well-known potential problem, often caused by a pacemaker left in the body being incinerated. These should be removed by the GP or undertaker beforehand and the cremation (or 'crem') forms require confirmation of this. One of these ovens had been damaged by the missed exploding pacemaker of our patient, but, thankfully, nobody else was hurt. I hope the noise was not too distressing for any mourners. The crematorium had two ovens but had to work at a reduced capacity for a short while afterwards while the damaged one was repaired.

Norman had missed the relevant 'pacemaker' sticker on the front of a patient's notes while filling in his portion of the crem form. I had nearly made the same mistake when another patient's notes had other papers clipped onto them, covering up the sticker. We changed the way that we recorded this information afterwards to try to minimise the risk of such a mistake ever happening again.

You Know When You Know, and I Knew

The GPs at my practice had traditionally retired at age sixty, and this had been my expectation, too, until I developed some serious health problems. The treatments and after-effects were having an impact on my comfort and concentration at work, so I realised that I would not be able to work full-time until the planned time. I had been toying with making The Decision for a few months, but felt too embarrassed and even guilty to discuss it with friends and colleagues. I was not used to giving up or giving in, so I decided to wait a bit longer.

Then I had a particularly stressful duty-day. By 10 a.m., I was feeling so much more overwhelmed than usual or expected that I started to compile a handwritten list of probable causes. By 7 p.m., as I was finishing up, my 'reasons to be hacked off' list had filled a page. Most of the items related to the numbers of inappropriately booked patients, extras and visits, as well as expanding piles of urgent paperwork and referrals. Oh, and I had forgotten my sandwich, although I'd had no time to eat it anyway.

I looked at the list, realising how ridiculous it, and maybe I, was. I knew then that the decision was made.

You know when you know, and I knew.

I got home an hour later and told Michelle that I was going to finish as soon as was sensible. This could not be very soon as I was a partner in the practice rather than being an employee. I told the practice manger the following day, and the GPs at our practice meeting the day after that. I gave just over twelve months' notice of my new retirement date, so that a replacement could be found. I then started to arrange things with the practice accountant and pensions people; I would take a small hit in my pension by taking it a year early but it would still be decent and manageable. Like many older GPs and hospital consultants, my pension savings were already being eaten into by recent tax changes, so that part was made slightly easier. I had already had to leave the pension scheme in order to try to minimise this impact: all a bit worrying in view of my serious health problems, as I was currently not covered by any NHS pension health or even death benefits for my family. These would be restored by actually taking my pension.

My partners and practice manager were kind enough to appear upset that I was leaving and soon started a provisional look around for my replacement. I prepared my colleague, Farzan, for her role in replacing me as senior partner, by telling her that there was no money attached to this role and the title simply meant that you were the oldest partner left standing. It also meant that she would simply have more responsibility and more paperwork to sign.

Lots more.

I felt better that The Decision was made and I could now ease down towards my retirement in twelve months.

Then came 2020.

The Year 2020 and
the Beginnings of Covid

January

The first few known cases in the UK were heavily reported from the end of January 2020 and these patients were generally kept at arm's length in quarantine. Sadly, it was already a bit late by then, as the disease had begun to spread in the UK, in part from Brits (including GPs) who had been skiing in Europe.

February

We start receiving communications from government and local health agencies about the forthcoming expected explosion in cases. It was still a bit hard to believe or accept that this could all really be coming here. One of our GPs, Dr Scott, was a bit more switched on with regard to national and local medical politics than the rest of us. In part, this was because he was the youngest, but also because he was actually just more switched on, to be fair. He told us of the discussions and fears haunting the higher echelons of government and health management that there could be upwards even of 500,000 deaths in the UK.

We were sent all kinds of protocols for managing folk who felt ill, primarily about trying to keep most people safe and well, but without exposing the other patients, and staff, to this deadly virus. Remembering, of course, that we had no access to any testing at that stage and also very little personal protective equipment (PPE). Even when the PPE started to arrive, it was clear that it was of insufficient quality and quantities to be able to cope. One of our receptionists brought in some suitable protective masks donated by her partner, who owned a garage. For a while these were the only safe masks we actually had in the surgery.

One of the key early messages was for us to try to keep infected patients out of our surgeries and us from seeing them at home. This effectively meant that the patients who most wanted to be seen face to face were the ones we were instructed to stay away from. This was a difficult balancing game to play. In the early days, I visited a number of patients (or their family members) who had denied any typical Covid symptoms, only to find them absolutely typical when I arrived and walked in to see the poor feverish patient coughing away.

We were informed by the government and our local clinical comissioning group (CCG) that we needed to switch to a total triage system at all GP surgeries. This meant that all appointments for GPs or nurses were to be initiated as a telephone (or video) call before a making a decision on whether the patient needed a home visit or a face-to-face appointment. Urgent and other time-important blood tests continued as normal in the surgery, with obvious space and time between patients for cleaning and ventilation. Childhood vaccinations continued as usual throughout, with longer intervals between patients, and patients waiting outside the building until they were called in.

In some areas, CCGs had arranged for a single central Covid hub for patients with significant or deteriorating symptoms to be assessed. The advantage with such a 'hot hub' system is that only one surgery or building in an area would be exposed to these patients with the presumed associated high risk of Covid infection. Only a few GPs and staff would also have to be exposed to this higher risk and need to wear the appropriate levels of PPE, if available. This would also minimise the risk to the rest of the, presumably non-Covid, patients who needed to come into the other GP surgeries. Our CCG was not interested in this model-of-care provision and asked all surgeries to see their own 'hot' patients. We therefore needed to rearrange our layout and throughput of patients to minimise risk of exposure of other patients and staff to infection, and to allow more sensible disinfection regimes. We even put up a small outbuilding to allow for better ventilation and separation from other patients, and also easier cleaning.

Many surgeries were already doing video consultations or internet/email consultations before the pandemic and embraced the changes a bit more enthusiastically than us initially, but it only took us a few days to make the switch to using videos, where necessary, and accepting picture messages when helpful. The biggest problem with this technology is that the patients most likely to have no access to a computer or smartphone are the patients who are most frequently the sickest: that is, the elderly, the confused or just bed-bound, very ill people.

(To be fair on the CCG, they instituted an excellent series of updates on appropriate good practice, together with algorithms to help manage patients by phone, online and also face to face. These continued until 2023, perhaps well after most people may have expected Covid to still be on their GPs' agenda.)

March

Early on, we had a gradual increase in telephone calls from patients with suspected Covid, and had many other calls about shielding and our services. Every day we were bombarded with more instructions and advice from the NHS and its various national and local agencies. We had daily practice meetings with GPs and our staff to try to adapt to the changes, both current and expected. There was a general feeling of impending doom. Overall, though, in the early days we were waiting with trepidation for the expected and overwhelming wave of illness to sweep across our area. It had the feel of a phoney war, akin to books and films I had read and seen about the beginning of World War II. Things gradually became busier and ramped up through spring and summer, but we were not as completely overwhelmed as was feared, in part, I am sure, due to the changes we had made. The ambulance and hospital services took, by far, the largest brunt of things.

Throughout the pandemic, we continued to see patients at home and in the surgery. I usually brought in four or more patients a day after phoning them first. At the time, and even now, I am aware of the outcry in the press and social media that many people felt that GPs were not doing any work or seeing any patients. That was certainly not the case in the surgeries I knew of locally, or in those of other colleagues and friends that I was aware of. There must be some truth in the claims, though. I recently read a book with diary entries from one GP who had added a chapter about coping with the pandemic in his surgery. It seemed that he had not seen a patient face to face for many months. I find it hard to see how that could have been safe for all of the patients who weren't seen and cannot accept that the triage at all the surgeries I am aware of was letting too many people to be seen.

Another role that GPs were allocated early on in the pandemic was to look through the records of all of their patients to see if they needed shielding. This was an immense task at very short notice, magnified by the fact that there were no clear guidelines. As more guidelines were issued by the government and specialists, we had to amend our advice to patients. Hundreds of patients were ringing every day to ask about the advice, which had implications for their work, travel and income. Many were understandably not happy with the advice given and tried to push us for change.

Some worthy shielders were worried that their new status would stop them from going on planned holidays, before events unfolded that would force most people to cancel holidays.

In contrast, many others who had conditions that were not high risk were contacting us and asking to be shielded.

. . .

Our first hospital-confirmed case was initially seen and examined in one of the GP's rooms. His symptoms had been atypical and he had no known risks of Covid exposure. We, much later, received confirmation of his diagnosis from the hospital, and extensive cleaning of the consulting and waiting rooms was undertaken. This gentleman was in ICU for over a month but survived and was discharged in reasonable health after two months.

As infections began to increase in the UK, the government's advisory teams were predicting an even higher number of infections and deaths: both on a mass scale. They opened several temporary emergency Nightingale hospitals to cope with potential increases in admissions and also provided extra temporary morgue space. The rules on death certification were temporarily relaxed by changes in the law, which were quickly pushed through Parliament. In addition, a new local visiting death-certification service was set up. This involved a 24-hour mobile GP team who would be able to visit and confirm deaths in the community; due to the legal changes, they would also be able to issue death certificates without even having previous knowledge of the patient. All of these changes showed the fear of an even larger loss of lives.

Our local CCG sent an email to all the GPs asking them to contact all 'frail' elderly patients living at home. This was in order to have a discussion on resuscitation, so that they would consider agreeing to, and then signing, a 'Do Not Resuscitate' form. The supposed purpose of this was to try to help avoid the ambulance service and hospital wards being overwhelmed by patients as they would be at very high risk of dying anyway.

I understood the need to try to protect and ration valuable resources to enable younger people, who were more likely to benefit, to have access to these potentially limited resources. I was not, however, happy to cold-call these patients and ask them to sign a form to exclude themselves from potentially curative medical care in such a way. I was adamant that this approach was inhumane and inappropriate, however well-intentioned. As a practice, we discussed and decided not to engage in this instruction. The idea of ringing people up, at a time when they could not access full GP services, to have a chat and ask them to give up their rights to emergency healthcare for a while, was abhorrent. This would also never be forgotten or forgiven by patients and their families. We continued to have sensible discussions on this delicate subject with all patients when appropriate to them at the time that they were being seen and reviewed, but certainly not in the manner proposed.

I understand that many GPs in our area and elsewhere did engage in ringing or writing to their frail and elderly patients about this matter, and this was passed on to the press by angry relatives, with understandable outcry.

It was unsurprising, but apparent quite early on, that doctors and nurses were among the high-risk groups for both catching and dying from Covid, especially in certain higher-risk groups. The NHS asked GPs to grade their relative risk to this disease based on ethnicity, health problems, age and weight. The idea was that the very highest-risk doctors may need to avoid face-to-face consultations, including home visits. Many of the GPs in our practice were borderline for this exclusion, but none actually crossed over. I was 5kg in weight away from a face-to-face ban, so teased my partners about going on an even higher-calorie diet to push me into the protected group. We would have struggled if we had all been in the higher-risk group as there was no available support for practices in that position. In the end, none of us ducked out of any duties due to our perceived risk, as this would have left our colleagues carrying a higher burden of work and risk.

The First Summer of Covid

Plenty of people in essential roles continued to leave the house and travel to work throughout the imposed lockdowns; these roles were numerous and spread far outside the NHS. We all know about shopworkers and the police and power company workers and sewage workers and lorry drivers and farmers and numerous other groups beyond that. Of course, other essential workers also continued to work from home if they were able to do so, and shielded people had to do the same if they were able. Many office-based workers were able to work from home and some people were furloughed.

I was lucky enough to live in a nice house with a nice garden, on a nice road in a nice middle-class commuter area. For several months during those lockdowns, it appeared that only a few people left our road to go to work, typically those of us working for the NHS, in hospital and GP roles. Several immediate neighbours had good professional roles in finance and banking and openly said how much they were enjoying not having to commute, instead working from home. I arrived home most evenings to find that they had been sunbathing and playing golf or mountain biking: this throughout that incredibly sunny spring and summer. Two of them told me it was the best year they had ever had, able to spend time with their children and close family and catch up on reading, and also learning to bake sourdough bread.

So far, so good, although I was obviously a bit envious. I was really, though, more irritated by their apparent ignorance of the troubles and trials of the rest of the population who did not have their advantages. A few of them also seemed oblivious to the severe nature of the pandemic, so far removed were they, in their leafy bubble, from the full impact of the disease and the lockdowns in the nearby towns and cities.

I was asked numerous times by neighbours, 'What do you think about this virus thing, then?'

This was usually followed by, 'I don't even know of anybody who has caught it, do you?'

I told them about the large number of patients and friends who had been, and were currently, ill, as well as the number of deaths. This information didn't seem to soak in very well, as they would ask me again a few weeks later, seemingly oblivious to our previous conversations.

During lockdown we needed a new boiler and associated repair work done in our house. Without exception, when any of the plumbers and other tradespeople found out what my work was, they asked me the same questions as my neighbours had. They all still seemed very doubtful and in denial about the pandemic, despite the news. It seemed that none of them had been directly touched or affected by the disease so, again, doubted the truth of it. All a bit odd, really, and the sign of worse to come with the torrents of misinformation that have now encouraged many people to become militant anti-vaxxers and conspiracy theorists.

Most of us haven't been to Australia, but we believe the people who have been, who tell us that there are kangaroos there. Especially when they show us the photographs and videos. There does seem to be an increasing anti-scientific bias to much of the information that people share on social media.

Many of the science doubters are also happy to believe that some scientists and designers of new phones and planes know their stuff, but think that medical scientists are covering up all the facts.

When the first hint of post-Covid syndrome, or long Covid, came along, it became apparent that there was no easy way of testing or confirming this diagnosis. It also appeared that many of those who had survived very severe illness with extended stays in intensive care units appeared to have escaped from major post-infective symptoms. Perhaps more surprisingly, many without definite proof of infection had persisting symptoms that were still likely to be due to Covid infection. This disparity in severity of the original illness, and the severity and longevity of presumed post-Covid symptoms, made it very difficult to accurately determine how much Covid itself was to blame for these symptoms.

There is also a great deal of symptom overlap between the milder symptoms and those of other post-viral fatigue conditions, and also with other physical or even depressive illnesses. The symptom list is long and varied, and many feel their lives have been completely taken over by them; the four main symptoms being insomnia, fatigue, breathlessness and anxiety. One of the other common long-term symptoms that are not seen as much after other viral illnesses is the complete loss of, or change in, sense of smell and taste. This can be very disturbing and have a great impact on somebody's quality of life, although thankfully usually resolves over time for most sufferers. At the moment, there does not appear to be any specific treatment for long Covid, with reliance being more on overall supportive care with the addition of a graduated exercise approach and added psychological support.

Gallows humour helps many of us to cope with stress, especially in the NHS. When awareness of long Covid hit the national news, we decided at the end of one of our practice meetings to select five names from our most regular attendees who we thought were the most likely to declare themselves as suffering from this dreadful condition. Four of these patients did indeed present, as predicted, all within a week. No doubt they genuinely felt ill and they were simply looking for a diagnosis to explain their chronic symptoms; nevertheless, it was predictable, literally, who would present first.

Time to Go

I had finished my evening surgery and was crossing the road at the traffic lights near to surgery, heading for my car. It had been a long day, during one of the Covid lockdowns. I had spent most of the day on telephone consultations, but had also done some home visits and seen a half-dozen patients, face to face, in the surgery.

A shout came from somebody in one of the cars that were stopped at the lights – 'Dr S!'

I shouted back towards the traffic, while still walking – 'Hi, are you OK?'

'No, we're not!' This time it was two voices in unison.

Then back to a single voice again – ''Cos we can't get an appointment with you!'

I still could not tell which car the voices were from, nor who had been shouting, as sunshine was reflecting from the car windscreens. I felt irritated at being shouted at in the street, but also guilty because they hadn't been able to get an appointment. It suddenly occurred to me, at that moment, that I was glad to be nearer the end than the beginning of my career.

I had continued to work as normal throughout the first eight months of the Covid pandemic before slipping out fairly quietly. The partners and staff bade me a more subdued farewell than we had expected, due to the rules in place at the time, but were really kind and I was lucky to still get a nice and thoughtful goodbye, with some lovely presents and an amazing bespoke cake. Sadly, I was unable to let all of our patients know about finishing, as we felt that this would be really tricky given the severe limitation on numbers of patients allowed into the surgery. I felt guilty about this, too, and I would have loved to say a proper goodbye to many of them, but things were difficult to say the least. Remember that families had been unable to see loved ones dying in hospital or even attend funerals in proper numbers.

Also, behind the scenes – and unknown to all but family and closest friends – I had developed a cardiac problem. The symptoms were starting to impact on my home and work life, and were getting much worse by the day. By my retirement day, I was struggling to even walk to my car, so it was a great relief when I finished.

Two weeks later, I underwent a cardiac procedure and was able to settle into a rehabilitation programme, in order to get, and hopefully stay, fitter. Thankfully, I had no symptoms after the treatment and just had to keep taking the tablets. There was no rush. I was now retired and had plenty of time to get better.

'Please Remove Your Jacket or Coat and Roll Up Your Sleeve'

Looking back, it is the memory of the car battery-charger packs in the health centre that perhaps sums up the Covid vaccine roll-out. With the lockdown came no use for cars. For many patients, it was their first trip out in months. Their cars had managed to get the patients to the health centre, but after the prescribed fifteen-minute wait (to ensure no adverse reaction to the jab), they found themselves unable to restart their engines.

Cue the need for battery restarting.

Two months into my retirement and recovery, I had begun the process of looking more seriously at some of my old hobbies that I had neglected for years.

I was settling into a bit of a routine until my partner, Michelle, and I were called for our first Covid vaccine at a drive-in centre. We spoke to some of my old former colleagues while we were there. It was made clear that they needed more helpers. Michelle offered to become a volunteer and I, slightly more reluctantly, agreed to do the same. We originally helped out at the drive-through vaccine clinics.

These often lasted eleven hours and were during many of the wettest and then the coldest days of the year. Sometimes I was lucky enough to work inside in the relative warm, but we were outside most of the time, even during heavy snowfall. Everything was thoughtfully organised and we were all well-fed at lunchtime, which was a great boost to morale. All of the paid and voluntary staff were well-motivated and pleased to be helping. The vast majority of patients were thrilled to be getting their jabs and just to be getting out, to be fair.

Our vaccine team later moved into a sports hall: doors open, no heating, but much more pleasant than being outside in the with zero-Celsius weather. Most of the team were the same, and spirits remained high. This was helped by the mood and attitude of the majority of the patients. At this stage, it was generally just the elderly and those with underlying medical conditions. Many of these were excited to get their vaccines and were loudly grateful. Many of the ladies cried with relief rather than fear or pain.

As the months went by, the ages of those being vaccinated became younger and younger, and the levels of appreciation and gratitude tended to fall with age, presumably as these patients were a bit less fearful of the virus and its potential consequences for them, personally. On many occasions, the queues to get into the centre were really quite long, and the level of complaints also increased in volume and frequency when we got to the younger age groups; by the time we were injecting the 16–18 year age groups, half of them would not even wait for the required fifteen-minute safe time after their Pfizer jabs.

Michelle's role as a volunteer was usually to check patients' booking details on the way into the hall, but also included cleaning chairs and checking patients' temperatures. Mine initially often tended to be similar general roles with some medical input. Over time I stepped up to being the medical clinical supervisor when the CCG vaccine lead GP was absent. I was therefore required to re-register with the GMC and undergo formal online training procedures again, like all the other clinical staff. I also had to 'learn' how to give vaccinations and be witnessed giving enough of these that I could be signed off as fit to do so. All this after over thirty-five years as a doctor.

The main star of the vaccine centre was the lead nurse, Belinda, who ran the floor area, supervising and giving vaccines. She also had the tendency to burst out into song-and-dance routines suddenly and unexpectedly. Many of the older patients often joined in, unembarrassed and laughing. Perhaps unsurprisingly, most of the younger patients and staff did not easily engage with these shenanigans, and tried to avoid eye contact with this uncool madwoman. She really lifted the spirits of the rest of us, especially on the longer shifts there, which often still lasted more than twelve hours. She was also marvellous when treating patients of any age who had special needs or learning difficulties: always kind, always patient.

Early on, the Pfizer vaccines had to be used within a few days once removed from the freezer. They were also too fragile to move to another centre once made up. The centre was not open every day, so this meant that we often had to stay a few hours later than expected, ringing around to try to find volunteers to come down for a jab and avoid unnecessary wastage. It was hard to gain full control over the numbers of vaccines needed to be defrosted and made up, as so many people did not turn up for their appointments. These being appointments that the patients had themselves booked over the previous week or so.

We often had up to 300 patients in a day not turn up. On other days, we had very few dropouts and hundreds of extra unbooked patients turned up, hopeful.

The vast majority of jabs were done in the sports hall, but the vaccine team also did all the jabs for the town's housebound patients, including those in old people's and nursing homes, as well as in pop-up clinics at local mosques, markets, colleges and even supermarkets. Attendances at the hall were high, with the team often vaccinating up to 1,800 people a day. Many of the patients had relevant medical questions and queries, so it was helpful for them to have a doctor there. Some days we also had a lot of patients fainting or panicking about fainting; they often required help from nurses or paramedics, and me.

The maximum number of fainters in a single day was eight.

As you may already know, fainting can be a bit catching, so many of these incidents often happened at almost the same time. This meant that there would sometimes be three people lying on the hall floor at a time, being tended to by staff and concerned relatives. Most were absolutely fine to leave after a short recovery time, with only a few needing any more prolonged treatment. Two required hospital transfer: one with persistent breathlessness and the other after sustaining a fractured wrist when he fainted outside.

A significant number of people initially refused to wear a mask when they came into the hall and some others claimed exemption on spurious health grounds. I generally have little sympathy for the majority of the anti-mask attendees at the centre, or even outside. There is, of course, the odd exception, particularly in people with severe learning impairments or psychological conditions who were disturbed by anything being put over their faces, and we did our best to accommodate them, even jabbing them outside or in cars.

Belinda was very good at persuading most of the others to just have a mask or alternative face shield for the required fifteen minutes or so; it was an NHS zone and some of the vulnerable people there were really anxious being inside with large numbers of people. In context, remember that all essential workers had been wearing face masks throughout their whole shifts, including, of course, the vaccine centre workers. Doctors, nurses and theatre technicians have always been required to wear masks for the whole of their time in operating theatres and I don't remember anybody ever objecting to this, or ever being asked how they felt about it.

One of the vaccine centre mask refuseniks later told me, ruefully, that he had bought his mask-exemption badge and certificate online.

Similarly, there were a fair share, too, of fervent anti-vaxxers, who turned up for an argument or just to disrupt things.

Some of the staff were threatened with violence in or outside the centre and the police needed to be called on a few occasions, but with only one arrest made during that time. Many other 'characters' turned up for jabs or even just discussions about the science or ethics of vaccinations; I'm not sure how many of these had previously challenged their routine vaccinations in the same manner.

I was a bit surprised to hear about the number of NHS clinical workers who had profound objections to compulsory Covid vaccinations, as vaccinations have been necessary for decades in most clinical roles. I don't recall anyone ever refusing to become a doctor, midwife or nurse because of this requirement to protect patients from specific infections. Thinking of hepatitis B, for instance, vaccination and boosters are compulsory for medics and failure of the jabs to raise the relevant antibodies in a given person is sufficient to require redeployment of that person into a less clinically involved position.

I was asked to speak to one chap who came into the centre.

'How can I help?' I said, sounding hopefully helpful.

'I came last week and they wouldn't give me a jab, 'cos I didn't have a GP.'

'Sorry about that. They actually could have done a jab for you in that case. They gave you the wrong information. Apologies.'

'Well, I wouldn't give them my name, either,' he volunteered.

'Why not?' I asked, now sensing a slightly awkward customer.

'Tax.'

'We are the NHS and don't pass any information to the tax authorities,' I said.

'Have you ever been to fuckin' prison?' he asked – rhetorically, I suspect.

Nevertheless I answered, albeit a bit snootily. 'No, of course I've never been to fuckin' prison. I'm a doctor.' (I know that, strictly speaking, I could have actually been to prison and still become a doctor, but I didn't feel it was the right time to get into that much detail.)

'Well, it's a fuckin' horrible place and I'm not going back.'

'I'm not sure what that's got to do with us giving you a jab,' I said, trying to get back on track.

'Well, I don't trust doctors, either. It took me six years to get a rash diagnosed when I was twelve. I demanded a second opinion.'

'Well, let's see if we can help you now. Have you registered with a GP?' I asked.

'Yeah.'

'And can we now have your name?'

'Yeah,' he said.

'OK, you can go and give your details to the girl over there and then she will show you to your seat.'

I was not quite sure why he wanted or needed to speak to me. I understand that he later got into an argument with the vaccinator about the jab he was having: preferring another brand. He eventually accepted the proffered one, then after being jabbed, walked straight out instead of waiting for the required time.

On another occasion, Belinda came over to tell me that a lady in her forties was asking if she could have a numbing gel on her arm before her vaccination. The answer was no, of course, but I suggested to Belinda that this lady was probably covered in tattoos. Belinda looked at me a little quizzically then walked back towards this lady. A few minutes later, she walked back over to me, shaking her head.

'How did you know she was covered in tattoos? Did you recognise her?' she asked.

'No, it's just that after thirty years in medicine, I've noticed that the only adults who tend to kick up a fuss about needles are the ones with lots of tattoos.' A sweeping statement, I know, but it was right on this occasion at least.

I worked at the vaccine centre for a year, into the booster programme; finishing when there was no longer a requirement for an on-site doctor.

And in the End

I was grateful for the opportunity that I was given to extend my medical career for this additional year, especially in a different and less stressful role. I had been feeling quite ill during my last few months of ordinary GP work, without realising quite how ill at the time. It was like only noticing how loud some background noise is when it suddenly stops and you wonder why you hadn't noticed it before.

It was also pointed out to me, by both Michelle and my old friend Mick, that I must have been glad to take retirement from GP work as I was obviously unhappy with it. I was surprised to hear this as didn't realise or think that I was, and even more surprised that it seemed apparent to others. Like most doctors (and teachers) I know, I think that I was in the habit of complaining and moaning about my work and workload so much that I probably had forgotten how much I still enjoyed many aspects of work.

I had always enjoyed trying to help people, particularly if they wanted genuine medical help. I enjoyed working with my great medical and nursing colleagues, and with the hardworking reception and admin staff, including a brilliant practice manager. They are still there, working hard and under pressure; the expectations of government and patients have changed so much over the years and the speed of these changes continues to increase exponentially. I feel some survivor's guilt for escaping in (almost) one piece.

Another thing that's stopped since I finished working are the regular work-anxiety dreams that I had for decades every Sunday night, in which I was either arriving at, or running late for, work.

These dreams often included scores of patients queuing outside my room, amid computer or technology failures. If I had been on leave for a week, I would also have the same dreams on the Saturday night as well as the Sunday.

Looking over the years, was it a good career choice, born as it was from the fortuitous crossing of paths with a medical student on an exchange trip?

Yes, of course it was, for me at least.

I think I was also reasonably good at the job, particularly communicating with and understanding patients, despite many of the funny misunderstandings offered in this book. I always tried to treat people as I would like others to treat me and my family. I was probably a bit too soft and non-confrontational with patients, until they crossed a red line: trying to manipulate or use me or our beloved health service.

Overall, I hope I made a positive difference to my patients' – and also colleagues' – lives. You might not think so from reading this memoir, as there are a few failed resuscitation attempts listed here. Over the years, several of our patients were actually in the more fortunate ten per cent group who survive in-surgery cardiac arrests thanks to successful resuscitation by our team, which also included me, on several occasions! In truth, lives lost are more easily seen and recorded, especially when they were lost in a dramatic or heartbreaking way, such as Jack's ('Last Words').

Lives saved are rarely seen in such a clear way as those lost. These are often prolonged by more gradual tweaks: appropriate recognition of disease and its proper treatment – often over many years, if you look at the use of preventative drugs, for example in high blood pressure or high cholesterol, or atrial fibrillation. Sometimes you just get a gut feeling when you are seeing a patient, particularly if you have got to know them well over time. When a patient who rarely complains, complains, you should pay attention. Both of these situations here are more easily managed when a patient is known to both you and the practice, and you have had time to establish a relationship. And mutual trust.

I would like to think that I used just enough humour in consultations to allow people to relax and feel comfortable, and that I always picked the right moments, too.

People still ask me, 'Don't you ever wish you'd been a specialist?'

The subtext and implication perhaps still being that only hospital doctors are proper doctors and that General Practice is some kind of refuge for the thick or unambitious, or those with a blood phobia.* Having, like all GPs, also worked in hospitals, I have the utmost respect for hospital doctors, junior and specialist. I know that most are extremely dedicated and continue to perform skilled work in extreme circumstances, as do most GPs, but ...

No.

The answer is no.

I think my interest in people and in communicating with – and also for – them, are the skills that I brought to the job. It felt right. It felt like I belonged there. It's been good, thanks.

Well, near the end may be good, but at the end is even better, so it's time to take the other Doc Martin's advice and stop speaking ...

---

*   Such as ITV's Doc Martin.

Postscript – What Next for General Practice?

The original and chief purpose of General Practice* was to be the first port of call for patients with symptoms and illnesses, and then to manage most of the revealed conditions: selecting who needs onward investigations or treatments in secondary care, before then managing them again after any clinic appointment or hospital admission.

Over the time I have worked in General Practice, numerous new tasks have been added to the overall workload, inevitably soaking up a substantial number of the available appointments. These include the longer-term management of most chronic diseases, which has already broadly moved from hospitals into General Practice, with even more planned to follow. Disease prevention has also been incorporated into the GP remit and now occupies a lot of GP time.

The average patient now attends the surgery for four times the number of appointments than they did in the 1980s. Many of these extra appointment slots are with other healthcare professionals rather than GPs, but are still often taken up with tasks that would formerly have been dealt with by GPs themselves.

---

* General Practice and GPs being used as a coverall, shorthand term in this chapter for the whole of the General Practice team, to avoid distraction and repetition. This usually includes nurses, nurse practitioners, advanced nurse practitioners, doctors in training, clinic room practitioners, managers, administration staff, pharmacists and receptionists, but can also include physiotherapists, paramedics, associate physicians/physician associates and others.

Even this expanded workforce seems unable to cope with the ever-increasing demand, which is far in excess of provision.

Innovations have been made to bridge the gap by adding different types of appointments such as telephone, video or online consultations; the roll-out of these technologies being accelerated by the pandemic. Very often these alternative appointments are actually more popular with younger patients, but sometimes less so with older patients, who tend to prefer the familiarity of a face-to-face appointment in the surgery.

The government has recently trumpeted an expansion in GP training places, but there is still a massive shortfall in actual hours of GP provision, as many of the newer recruits work part-time. So hard is it to replace retired doctors that many surgeries, especially in more deprived areas, have closed for good, adding to the demand at other local surgeries. Decreasing numbers of young trainees are willing to commit to the old-style standard GP career: that is, being a partner in a practice from their late twenties through to retirement at sixty, or thereabouts.

As an example, during my last year in my local GP training group, only three of the thirty-plus GP trainees expressed any intention to work as a GP and only one of these three intended to stay in the area, and he only wanted to work part-time from day one.

These trainees were mostly at the end of their five-year postgraduate training, three years of it having been focused on General Practice, with nearly two years of that time actually working in GP surgeries.

It is not clear why most of them no longer want to pursue their planned career path. There is possibly the unwillingness of younger people to commit to a lifetime of responsibility at one place, added to the current wide availability of alternative employment in out-of-hours and walk-in centres; but we have to face the fact that they have seen General Practice, warts and all (literally), and just don't like it.

There are many different approaches to fill the gap in front-line practitioners by employing other qualified staff in that position. Recently, ambulance paramedics have been successfully employed by practices in a triaging or visiting role, but they are not usually trained to deal with the management of longer-term physical or mental health complaints.

Another attempt to plug the care gaps left by failing GP numbers has been the importation and adoption of an idea from the USA: that of physician associates, a.k.a. associate physicians (PAs or APs). These are (usually) science graduates who have then undergone a further two years of university-based training. The idea is that they can then sit in GPs' surgeries (or other NHS settings) and interview patients before feeding back to doctors. They cannot prescribe, nor order X-rays or CT scans, but can manage longer-term conditions in patients and also health promotion. I am a little cynical about this particular role, as so many of these patients still need further GP input, and I don't feel that two years of medical training should be sufficient to allow them to use physician in their title. This in itself is a bit confusing for patients; one of my family members was booked in for such an appointment and was led to believe that the practitioner was some kind of more qualified doctor – being an associate, after all. All this while partially competing with doctors who have previously undergone ten years minimum of training. PAs are, of course, paid a lot less, so therein also lies some of the pull of this type of stopgap. A recent TV documentary has exposed the overuse of PAs in many UK GP practices owned by an American company. An example was given of one practice, which had six PAs and no actual GPs present on the premises, at any time. Potentially very lucrative and dangerous at the same time, and certainly not a good practice to be a patient at.

Are there any obvious solutions to the workforce crisis?

Putting more money into GP services is an obvious and predictable answer and would certainly help, but I am not sure that this would automatically solve all of the problems of General Practice recruitment and retention. I note that the government has recently announced an expansion of medical school places and also shortening the course to four years, although the BMA appears wary of the possible consequences of under-training doctors; hard as it is to imagine what can be left out of the current curriculum.

Another, more sustainable, approach in the longer term would be to trust the frontline staff to manage available resources more, as they usually know what the needs and likely solutions are for their area, with some safeguarding in place, naturally, for patients and precious NHS funds. Empowering people with the ability to change and improve things in this way has the tendency to raise morale in the workforce and encourages them to continue the good work, eventually leading to enhancing medical and nursing recruitment and retention.

To some extent, the roll-out of more localised decision-making groups in General Practice has already started and is already being enhanced by the increasingly active role planned for primary care networks (PCNs). Let's hope that they are allowed to achieve some genuine changes before yet another NHS structural management reshuffle takes place.

We can all hark back to the imagined glory days of General Practice and the NHS, generally, of old, perhaps forgetting that things were far from perfect then, too. Our parents and grand-parents who had been raised in a more austere world would often put up with all kinds of pain and misery to avoid being a trouble to anyone else.

We all expect more now.

So we should.

General Practice can still offer a great service in the future. It just needs the right financial resources and to be allowed some independence in managing local healthcare needs. It is still full of bright, hard-working, problem-solving doctors and their colleagues, all of whom want the best for their patients and communities.

Trust me, as the saying goes.

Acknowledgements

I would like to take this opportunity to thank:

Michelle, for her patience and practical support while I was writing this book.

Oh yes, and also for marrying me last summer!

The team at Whitefox for their guidance and professionalism, with special thanks to John Bond and Rosie Pearce. Thanks also to Jemima Hunt for directing me towards them in the first place and then for her thoughtful and objective editing.

My friends Mike, Steve and Jane for all of their interest and encouragement.

All of my other friends and colleagues in my old practice, many of them still hard at work in the surgery. It is difficult to thank you properly while still allowing you the relative anonymity that is needed. You all know how hard and thankless it can be in general practice, but still fight to do an amazing job.

Mostly to all of the patients that I had the honour of treating over the years. I tried my best and hope that I got a lot more right than I got wrong. Thank you for sharing some of your difficult times with me, as well as the funny and unusual ones.

Lastly, thanks to the BBC for the inspirational *The Body in Question* series by Dr Jonathan Miller; the fictional, but intently realistic, *Cardiac Arrest* series by Jed Mercurio; and for originally showing *M*A*S*H*, featuring Hawkeye, of course.